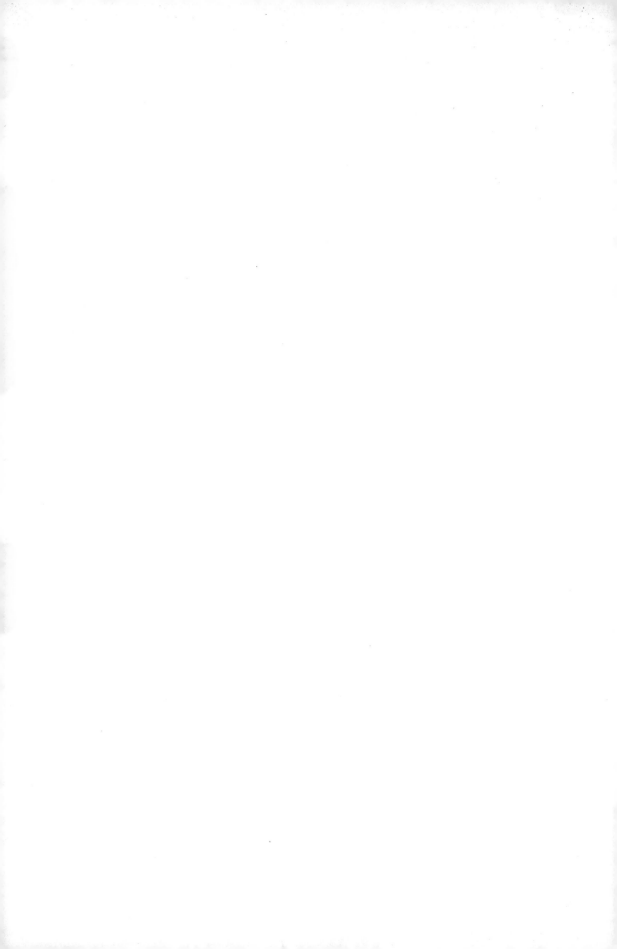

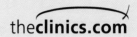
theclinics.com

PET CLINICS

Lung Cancer

Guest Editor
JAMES W. FLETCHER, MD

October 2006 • Volume 1 • Number 4

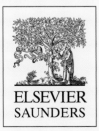
ELSEVIER
SAUNDERS

An imprint of Elsevier, Inc
PHILADELPHIA LONDON TORONTO MONTREAL SYDNEY TOKYO

W.B. SAUNDERS COMPANY

A Division of Elsevier Inc.

1600 John I: Kennedy Boulevard • Suite 1800 • Philadelphia, Pennsylvania 19103-2899

http://www.theclinics.com

PET CLINICS Volume 1, Number 4

October 2006 ISSN 1556-8598, ISBN 1-4160-3935-X

Editor: Barton Dudlick

Reprints: For copies of 100 or more, of articles in this publication, please contact the commercial Reprints Department, Elsevier Inc., 360 Park Avenue South, New York, New York 10010-1710. Tel.: (+1) 212-633-3813; Fax: (+1) 212-462-1935; E-mail: reprints@elsevier.com

The ideas and opinions expressed in *PET Clinics* do not necessarily reflect those of the Publisher. The Publisher does not assume any responsibility for any injury and/or damage to person or property arising out of or related to any use of the material contained in this periodical. The reader is advised to check the appropriate medical literature and the product information currently provided by the manufacturer of each drug to be administered to verify the dosage, the method and duration of administration, or contraindications. It is the responsibility of the treating physician or other health care professional, relying on independent experience and knowledge of the patient, to determine durg dosages and the best treatment for the patient. Mention of any product in this issue should not be construed as endorsement by the contributors, editors, or the Publisher of the product or manufactureers' claims.

PET Clinics (ISSN 1556-8598) is published quarterly by W.B. Saunders, 360 Park Avenue South, New York, NY 10010-1710. Months of publication are January, April, July, and October. Business and Editorial Offices: 1600 John F. Kennedy Blvd., Suite 1800, Philadelphia, PA 19103-2899. Accounting and Circulation Offices: 6277 Sea Harbor Drive, Orlando, FL 32887-4800. Periodicals postage paid at New York, NY, and additional mailing offices. Subscription prices are USD 180 per year for US individuals, USD 223 per year for US institutions, USD 81 per year for US students and residents, USD 184 per year for Canadian individuals, USD 212 per year for Canadian institutions, USD 180 per year for international individuals, USD 244 per year for international institutions and USD 92 per year for Canadian and foreign students/residents. To receive student and resident rate, orders must be accompanied by name of affiliated institution, date of term, and the signature of program/residency coordinator on institution letterhead. Orders will be billed at individual rate until proof of status is received. Foreign air speed delivery is included in all Clinics subscription prices. All prices are subject to change without notice. POSTMASTER: Send address changes to *PET Clinics*, Elsevier Periodicals Customer Service, 6277 Sea Harbor Drive, Orlando, FL 32887-4800. **Customer service: 1-800-654-2452 (US). From outside of the US, call (+1) 407-345-4000.**

Printed in the United States of America.

LUNG CANCER

MICHAEL P. MAC MANUS, MD, MRCP, FRCR, FFRRCSI, FRANZCR
Associate Professor, Department of Radiation Oncology, Peter MacCallum Cancer Centre, East Melbourne, Victoria, Australia

SANDRA J. ROSENBAUM, MD
Department of Nuclear Medicine, University of Duisburg, Essen, Germany

EGBERT F. SMIT, MD, PhD
Professor of Pulmonology, Department of Pulmonary Diseases, VU University Medical Center, Amsterdam, The Netherlands

SIGRID STROOBANTS, MD, PhD
PET Center (Nuclear Medicine), University Hospital Gasthuisberg, Catholic University, Leuven, Belgium

SHAWN D. TEAGUE, MD
Assistant Professor of Radiology, Department of Radiology, Indiana University School of Medicine, Indianapolis, Indiana

JOHAN VANSTEENKISTE, MD, PhD
Respiratory Oncology Unit (Pulmonology), Leuven Lung Cancer Group, University Hospital Gasthuisberg, Catholic University, Leuven, Belgium

HARM VAN TINTEREN, MSc
Statistician, Comprehensive Cancer Center, Amsterdam, The Netherlands

JOKKE WYNANTS, MD
Respiratory Oncology Unit (Pulmonology), Leuven Lung Cancer Group, University Hospital Gasthuisberg, Catholic University, Leuven, Belgium

LUNG CANCER

Volume 1 · Number 4 · October 2006

Contents

A solitary pulmonary nodule, which is defined as less than 3 cm in diameter, is a common incidental finding on routine radiographic imaging. Early diagnosis is important for the treatment of malignancies. Radiologic assessment can evaluate many characteristics such as size, margin, contour, and internal characteristics to predict if a lesion is benign or malignant. In this article, the assessment of a solitary pulmonary nodule using radiographic features is reviewed.

Imaging techniques play a vital role in the diagnosis, staging, and follow-up of patients who have lung cancer. For this purpose, PET has become an important adjunct to conventional imaging techniques such as chest radiography, CT, ultrasonography, and MR imaging. The ability of PET to differentiate the metabolic properties of tissues allows more accurate assessment of undetermined lung lesions, mediastinal lymph nodes, or extrathoracic abnormalities, tumor response after induction treatment, and detection of disease recurrence.

The superiority of PET imaging to structural imaging in many cancers is rapidly transforming the practice of radiotherapy planning, especially in lung cancer. Although most lung cancers are potentially treatable with radiation therapy, only patients who have truly locoregionally confined disease can be cured by this modality. PET improves selection for high-dose radiation therapy by excluding many patients who have incurable distant metastasis or extensive locoregional spread. In those patients suitable for definitive treatment, PET can help shape the treatment fields to avoid geographic miss and minimize unnecessary irradiation of normal tissues. PET will allow for more accurately targeted dose escalation studies in the future and could potentially lead to better long-term survival.

GOAL STATEMENT

The goal of the *PET Clinics* is to keep practicing radiologists and radiology residents up to date with current clinical practice in positron emission tomography by providing timely articles reviewing the state of the art in patient care.

ACCREDITATION

PET Clinics is planned and implemented in accordance with the Essential Areas and Policies of the Accreditation Council for Continuing Medical Education (ACCME) through the joint sponsorship of the University of Virginia School of Medicine and Elsevier. The University of Virginia School of Medicine is accredited by the ACCME to provide continuing medical education for physicians.

The University of Virginia School of Medicine designates this educational activity for a maximum of 60 *AMA PRA Category 1 Credits*™. Physicians should only claim credit commensurate with the extent of their participation in the activity.

The American Medical Association has determined that physicians not licensed in the US who participate in this CME activity are eligible for *AMA PRA Category 1 Credits*™.

Credit can be earned by reading the text material, taking the CME examination online at http://www.theclinics.com/home/cme, and completing the evaluation. After taking the test, you will be required to review any and all incorrect answers. Following completion of the test and evaluation, your credit will be awarded and you may print your certificate.

FACULTY DISCLOSURE/CONFLICT OF INTEREST

The University of Virginia School of Medicine, as an ACCME accredited provider, endorses and strives to comply with the Accreditation Council for Continuing Medical Education (ACCME) Standards of Commercial Support, Commonwealth of Virginia statutes, University of Virginia policies and procedures, and associated federal and private regulations and guidelines on the need for disclosure and monitoring of proprietary and financial interests that may affect the scientific integrity and balance of content delivered in continuing medical education activities under our auspices.

The University of Virginia School of Medicine requires that all CME activities accredited through this institution be developed independently and be scientifically rigorous, balanced and objective in the presentation/discussion of its content, theories and practices.

All authors/editors participating in an accredited CME activity are expected to disclose to the readers relevant financial relationships with commercial entities occurring within the past 12 months (such as grants or research support, employee, consultant, stock holder, member of speakers bureau, etc.). The University of Virginia School of Medicine will employ appropriate mechanisms to resolve potential conflicts of interest to maintain the standards of fair and balanced education to the reader. Questions about specific strategies can be directed to the Office of Continuing Medical Education, University of Virginia School of Medicine, Charlottesville, Virginia.

The authors/editors listed below have identified no professional or financial affiliations for themselves or their spouse/partner:
Gerald Antoch, MD; Andreas Bockisch, MD, PhD; Dewey J. Conces, Jr., MD; Christophe Dooms , MD; Barton Dudlick (Acquisitions Editor); James W. Fletcher, MD (Guest Editor); Lutz Stefan Freudenberg, MD, MA, MBA; Rodney J. Hicks, MD, FRACP; Otto S. Hoekstra, MD, PhD; Michael P. Mac Manus, MD, MRCP, FRCR, FFRRCSI, FRANZCR; Sandra Julie Rosenbaum, MD; Egbert F. Smit, MD, PhD; Sigrid Stroobants , MD, PhD; Johan Vansteenkiste, MD, PhD; Harm van Tinteren, MSc; and, Jokke Wynants, MD.

The authors/editors listed below identified the following professional or financial affiliations for themselves or their spouse/partner:
Thomas Beyer, PhD is employed by Timaq Medical Imaging Inc.
Michael K. Gould, MD, MS spouse is employed by Genentech, Inc.
Shawn D. Teague, MD is a consultant for Philips Medical Systems.

Disclosure of Discussion of non-FDA approved uses for pharmaceutical products and/or medical devices:
The University of Virginia School of Medicine, as an ACCME provider, requires that all faculty presenters identify and disclose any "off label" uses for pharmaceutical and medical device products. The University of Virginia School of Medicine recommends that each physician fully review all the available data on new products or procedures prior to instituting them with patients.

TO ENROLL

To enroll in the PET Clinics Continuing Medical Education program, call customer service at 1-800-654-2452 or visit us online at www.theclinics.com/home/cme. The CME program is available to subscribers for an additional fee of $175.00.

POSITRON
EMISSION
TOMOGRAPHY

PET Clin 1 (2006) ix–x

ELSEVIER
SAUNDERS

Preface

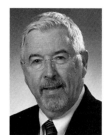

James W. Fletcher, MD
Guest Editor

James W. Fletcher, MD
Division of Nuclear Medicine
PET Imaging Center
Department of Radiology
Indiana University School of Medicine
Indiana/Purdue University at Indianapolis University
Hospital, Room 0655
550 North University Boulevard
Indianapolis, IN 46234, USA

E-mail address:
jwfletch@iupui.edu

Positron emission tomography (PET) is now an important cancer-imaging tool, both for diagnosis and staging, as well as offering prognostic information based on response. PET is the gold standard in the evaluation of an indeterminate solitary pulmonary nodule (SPN) or mass, where PET has proved to be significantly more accurate than computed tomography (CT). PET is significantly more accurate than CT in the evaluation of metastatic spread to locoregional lymph nodes, so that invasive surgical staging may be omitted in many patients with negative mediastinal PET images. Invasive surgical staging remains mandatory in patients with positive mediastinal PET images because of the possibility of false-positive findings owing to inflammatory nodes or granulomatous disorders. PET is a useful adjunct to conventional imaging in the search for metastatic spread. This may be due to the finding of unexpected metastatic lesions or the exclusion of malignancy in lesions that are equivocal on standard imaging. However, at this time, PET does not replace conventional imaging.

The evaluation of SPNs was one of the first Centers for Medicare and Medicaid Services approved and widespread Fluorodeoxyglucose-PET oncologic applications. Collectively, more has been published on the use of FDG-PET in evaluation of SPNs and staging of non–small-cell lung cancer (NSCLC) than any other clinical PET application. The evaluation of lung cancer probably represents the most common application of FDG-PET in most clinical departments.

Lung cancer is currently the leading cause of cancer deaths among both men and women in the United States, with statistical estimates of 169,400 new diagnoses and 154,900 cancer deaths in 2002.

In editing this issue of *Positron Emission Tomography Clinics* on lung cancer, I have endeavored to incorporate the perspectives of a number of specialists who are typically involved in the diagnosis, treatment, and management of patients with lung cancer. Contributions are presented from the perspective of the pulmonary radiologist, the interventional radiologist, the respiratory medical oncologist, the radiation therapy oncologist, and

doi:10.1016/j.cpet.2007.01.001

nuclear medicine/PET specialists. Two articles were written by individuals who have special additional expertise and experience in medical economics and cost–benefit, cost-effectiveness analysis (CEA).

The article on the diagnosis of lung cancer from the perspective of the pulmonary radiologist is presented by Drs. Teague and Conces. This article is a superb summary of the radiographic features of lung cancer that is very well illustrated with excellent examples of the radiographic features of both benign and malignant nodules and masses. The roles of transthoracic needle biopsy and bronchoscopic biopsy are also discussed.

In their article on staging of lung cancer, Drs. Wynants et al. provide an excellent overview of lung cancer staging as well as detailed information on the N-, T-, and M-factors. They also discuss the impact of FDG-PET in the workup of lung cancer, with emphasis on the valuable role of PET in guidance for invasive procedures. An example of the beneficial impact of PET on overall stage and patient management is the substantial reduction in the number of futile thoracotomies observed when PET is incorporated into the workup.

Dr. Michael Mac Manus provides an entire article devoted to the role of PET in radiation therapy planning. He presents a detailed summary and review of the role of imaging in radiation oncology, with special emphasis on PET and PET/CT. The results of the use of PET for selection of patients for radical radiation therapy and the impact of PET on patient outcomes are also discussed. It is clear that PET is transforming the way that radiation oncologists approach the treatment of lung cancer. The use of PET for selection of patients for radical therapy alone has already improved the apparent success rate with radiation therapy.

In the first article on the cost-effectiveness of FDG-PET, Drs. Hoekstra et al. detail their experience with the introduction of PET in the Netherlands, together with the design of parallel cost-effectiveness studies from their institution and other hospitals in their region. Techniques and designs for decision modeling and clinical value studies are described in detail, along with the intrinsic problems of implementation. The authors define reason-able outcome measures for randomized clinical trials (RCTs) that employ diagnostic imaging procedures, ie, the extent to which appropriate therapy is applied as a result of the diagnostic intervention. The results of their PET in lung cancer staging (PLUS) multicenter study are presented as an example of a well-designed RCT with FDG-PET as the imaging modality, where the use of PET resulted in a 50% reduction in futile thoracotomies.

A more specific example of cost-effectiveness studies in imaging is presented in an article on the cost-effectiveness of PET for characterizing SPNs by Dr. Michael Gould. This article introduces the topic of CEA with a very clear and understandable discussion of CEA compared with other types of economic evaluations. The author also provides the reader with a concise guide to interpreting the results of a CEA. The results of several CEA studies on FDG-PET in SPN are reviewed, with comments and critiques regarding strengths and weaknesses of study design. As the author points out, payers will likely require evidence of cost-effectiveness when making future coverage decisions as health care costs continue to increase in this country.

An important treatise on the accuracy of dual-modality FDG-PET/CT imaging in the staging of NSCLC compared with FDG-PET alone, as well as FDG-PET and CT read side by side, is presented in the article on anato-metabolic imaging by Drs. Freudenberg et al. These authors discuss the value and limitations of software versus hardware imaging fusion in FDG-PET/CT. The results of several recent large studies indicate a definite advantage for hardware dual-modality imaging fusion, inasmuch as the combined modality is able to detect significantly more lesions and has a larger impact on change/modification of patient management. As a bonus, the article provides the reader with an excellent summary of features designed to optimize FDG-PET/CT imaging protocols.

Many thanks are extended to all of the authors who contributed to this issue of *Positron Emission Tomography Clinics* for their diligence and support.

A variation on the ancient Chinese proverb/curse is offered to all: "May we continue to live in interesting times."

POSITRON
EMISSION
TOMOGRAPHY

PET Clin 1 (2006) 289–300

ELSEVIER
SAUNDERS

Diagnosis of Lung Cancer: Perspective of a Pulmonary Radiologist

Shawn D. Teague, MD*, Dewey J. Conces, Jr, MD

- Clinical
- Radiography
- Location
- Number
- Size
- Calcification
- Dynamic enhancement
- Attenuation

- Morphology
- Margin
- Cavitation
- Growth rate
- Bayesian analysis
- Follow-up
- Tissue diagnosis
- References

The solitary pulmonary nodule (SPN), a common incidental finding on routine radiographic imaging, is defined as a focal, oval, or round area of increased density in the lung that is less than 3 cm in diameter. In fact, there are an estimated 150,000 SPNs detected annually in the United States [1], and a single pulmonary nodule is detected on up to 0.2% of all chest radiographs [2]. The majority of SPNs are due to benign diseases such as hamartomas or granulomas [3,4]. A significant number, however, are malignant (up to 40% of single pulmonary nodules) [5]. Because the care of lung cancer is dependent on diagnosis at an early stage, it is important to evaluate nodules as expeditiously as possible. The evaluation of an SPN involves the use of a variety of modalities, because up to 25% to 39% of malignant nodules are inaccurately classified as benign after radiologic assessment of size, margin, contour, and internal characteristics [6]. In this article, the authors address the assessment of SPN radiographically for benign or malignant characteristics.

Clinical

Patient history plays a significant role in the evaluation of SPNs. A patient under 30 years old has a very low risk of an SPN being malignant unless the patient has a known extrathoracic malignancy. As the age of the patient increases, the likelihood of malignancy tends to increase.

There are other risk factors that significantly increase the likelihood of malignancy, such as a history of smoking, asbestos exposure, coal mining occupation, fibrosis, and known extrathoracic malignancy. In a patient who has a history of smoking, the incidence of lung cancer no longer increases once the patient ceases to smoke; however, the incidence is never equal to that of an individual who has never smoked. Presenting symptoms can be an important factor from a clinical standpoint in determining the likelihood of malignancy. In a patient who has suspected infection, it is reasonable to pursue a less aggressive course and obtain

Department of Radiology, Indiana University School of Medicine, 550 North University Boulevard, Room 0279, University Hospital, Indianapolis, IN 46250, USA
* Corresponding author.
E-mail address: sdteague@iupui.edu (S.D. Teague).

1556-8598/07/$ – see front matter © 2007 Elsevier Inc. All rights reserved.
pet.theclinics.com

doi:10.1016/j.cpet.2006.09.004

short-term follow-up radiographic imaging to document improvement in the nodule. In certain extrathoracic primary malignancies, the risk of an SPN being a metastases is much greater (such as melanoma, sarcoma, or testicular carcinoma) compared with other malignancies (such as head and neck squamous cell carcinoma) in which an SPN is much more likely to be a primary lung malignancy [7].

Radiography

The first imaging usually performed is the plain chest radiograph. An SPN, however, is seldom noted on a chest radiograph before it reaches 9 mm in diameter [8]. The false-negative rate for primary lung cancer on routine radiographic examinations has been reported to be 30% to 40% [9]. When evaluating plain radiographs, it is important to obtain prior examinations for comparison. A multicenter trial from the Mayo Clinic indicated that nearly 90% of peripheral lung cancers could be seen retrospectively on prior radiographic examination that were reported as negative at the time of initial interpretation [10]. Missed or overlooked lung nodules tend to occur in the lung apices, perihilar regions, and behind the heart and diaphragm on the frontal view. On the lateral view, lesions are typically missed when located posteriorly over the spine or anteriorly over the heart [11,12].

Some lesions can be determined as benign on a plain radiograph; however, most lesions will require further evaluation. If there is a question that the density seen on a chest radiograph represents a real nodule, chest fluoroscopy can be performed. Fluoroscopy can be used to determine if the nodule is real and not just an overlap of other soft tissues resulting in a "pseudonodule." Up to 20% of suspected nodules are actually mimics of other entities such as rib fractures, skin lesions, or combined areas of soft tissue attenuation [1]. Low kilovolts peak chest radiographs can be obtained to determine if calcification is present.

If these two examinations are not performed or are nonconclusive, the next diagnostic imaging test to consider is a thoracic CT examination. This examination cannot only define the morphologic characteristics of the nodule, but excels at identification of calcification within the nodule. CT is 10 to 20 times more sensitive for calcification when compared with traditional tomography, and 22% to 36% of nodules not obviously calcified on tomograms are shown to contain calcification on CT examination [13–15]. CT also allows quantitative assessment of calcification present in the nodule [15–18]. If the calcification is visible on thin-

section CT images, the Hounsfield measurement will usually have values of 400 H or greater. However, calcium can be present and not grossly visible. Therefore, if the measurement is 200 H or greater, then the nodule can be declared as containing calcification [19]. CT can also further characterize the features of the nodule, including nodule margin, tissue composition, number and size of lesions, and growth rate (when serial examinations are available). However, nodules can also be missed on CT scans. Swensen and colleagues [20] reported that of nodules that were missed on previous screening CT examinations, 62% were less than 4 mm in diameter, 37% were between 4 mm and 7 mm, and 2% were 8 mm to 20 mm in diameter. Ko and colleagues [21] reported that ground glass nodules were less frequently detected (65%) compared with solid nodules (83%) and there was a decreased sensitivity for detecting central compared with peripheral nodules (61% versus 80%). Finally, they also reported nodules adjacent to the pleura were better detected (84%) versus those not in contact with the pleural surface (75%).

Thinner sections, multiplanar reformats (especially MIPs), and cine viewing have all been shown to improve nodule detection [22–25]. CAD systems are being developed to help improve the nodule detection on both plain radiography and CT examinations. The efficiency of CAD systems has been reported to be between 38% and 95% [21].

The CT evaluation of a patient who has proven or suspected SPN should start with an examination without use of intravenous contrast through the entire chest. This serves to locate the nodule for further evaluation with thin sections, and also to document other abnormalities that include effusions, lymphadenopathy, or additional nodules. If there is only an SPN, then thin-section (1–3 mm) CT examination is suggested to fully characterize an SPN. Unless characteristics such as central calcification or fat are noted, the nodule will still remain indeterminate. In this situation, the nodule can be further evaluated with dynamic contrast-enhanced CT scan if it meets the appropriate criteria, or followed up over time with serial CT scans for growth assessment. Those nodules with characteristics suggesting malignancy can be further evaluated with a radiographic or surgical biopsy procedure.

With multidetector CT scanners, the thoracic scans can be performed with isotropic images retrospectively reconstructed from the raw data of routine helical scans provided the thinnest detector configuration is used for the initial routine scan. This somewhat eliminates the need to obtain additional thin sections specifically through the nodule in question. These thin sections are also useful for analysis by CAD programs and for performing computer-based lung nodule volume assessment.

Location

The location of an SPN can have some predictive value of the likelihood for malignancy. For example, lung cancer is 1.5 times more common in the right lung compared with the left lung, and 70% of lung cancers are in the upper lobes [26,27]. In patients who have pulmonary fibrosis, lung cancers are more likely in the periphery of the lower lobes [28]. Squamous cell carcinomas are more likely to present centrally, whereas about half of adenocarcinomas are peripheral in location [29].

Number

Multiple lung nodules are often found when performing CT on a patient suspected of having only an SPN that is based on plain film evaluation. Multiple nodules are more suggestive of previous granulomatous disease or metastatic disease. If one nodule is more dominant, it might be a solitary malignancy in the presence of other benign lesions such as granulomas. If two nodules are found, there is a chance both nodules could be primary lung cancer occurring synchronously, and both may be resectable; however, this occurs in less than 1% of patients [30,31].

The presence of satellite lesions, small nodules associated with a large dominant nodule, is suggestive of a benign etiology and usually indicative of granulomatous disease. The positive predictive value for these lesions is approximately 90% [32].

Size

Smaller lesions have a much higher likelihood of being benign. In fact, 80% of benign nodules are smaller than 2 cm in diameter [32–34]. However, malignant lesions can be small in size as well, with 15% of malignant nodules being less than 1 cm in diameter, and 42% being less than 2 cm in diameter [15,18,35].

Calcification

Lesions that are less than 9 mm in diameter noted on chest radiographs are likely diffusely calcified and are therefore benign (Fig. 1). As nodules become larger in diameter, the certainty of calcification becomes more difficult on plain radiography (Fig. 2). The sensitivity and specificity of reliably detecting calcification in one study where the nodules had a mean diameter of 13 mm was 50% and 87%, respectively [36].

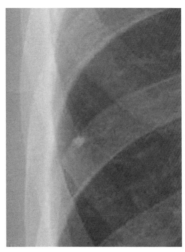

Fig. 1. Small right lung nodule that is very dense for its size, indicating it is calcified.

Patterns of nodule calcification include central, laminar/concentric, diffuse, popcorn, stippled, and eccentric. The most useful calcification patterns are central, laminated, or diffuse calcifications, which virtually exclude the likelihood of malignancy (Fig. 3) [37]. These patterns of calcification are typically associated with prior infection. Histoplasmosis, which is common in the Ohio River Valley, and tuberculosis are the two most common infectious diseases that demonstrate calcified benign appearing pulmonary nodules [1]. The popcorn pattern of calcification is characteristic of chondroid calcification seen in hamartomas (Fig. 4) [1]. When these particular patterns of calcification are present, they are reliable indicators of a benign nodule. However, 38% to 63% of benign nodules do not contain calcification, and even in hamartomas the reported prevalence of calcification is 5% to 50% [38–40].

Sometimes a malignant lesion such as an adenocarcinoma may grow to incorporate a granuloma, which is calcified (Fig. 5). However, this calcification when incorporated into the malignant lesion will almost certainly be eccentric in location [37]. Eccentric calcification is indeterminate, because a benign lesion may sometimes calcify in an eccentric pattern as well.

Bronchogenic carcinomas can show small flecks of calcification in up to 10% of tumors; however, this appears as a stippled pattern and is not usually detectable at radiographic evaluation [37]. Therefore, a small central calcification should be considered insufficient to make a diagnosis of a benign nodule. A stippled pattern can also be seen in metastases from mucin-secreting tumors such as colon or ovarian malignancies. Up to one third of carcinoid tumors may demonstrate calcification on

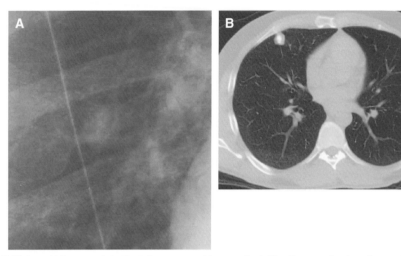

Fig. 2. (*A*) Right mid-lung nodule that shows no evidence of calcification on chest radiograph. (*B*) CT scan of the nodule demonstrating dense central calcification.

CT examination [1]. In lung cancer, calcification can be seen in up to 6% of cases on CT evaluation with the calcification usually being diffuse and amorphous [41].

Certain metastatic malignant lesions may contain calcification such as metastatic bone tumors (ie, osteosarcoma). Therefore, in patients who have known bone tumors, evaluation of lung nodules for calcification should be performed with great care to prevent misdiagnosis of a calcified metastatic lesion as a benign nodule.

Dynamic enhancement

In general, carcinomas enhance more after the administration of intravenous contrast than do benign nodules. Enhancement of less than 15 H has been shown to have a 96% negative predictive value for malignancy. However, the positive predictive value (68%) [26] is not nearly as strong because there can be many benign lesions that demonstrate enhancement mostly related to active inflammation. Lesions less than 8 mm in diameter, cavitary, or with central necrosis are not amenable to CT enhancement studies [26,42,43]. There are some data that suggest blood flow within a malignant nodule is quantitatively and qualitatively different than a benign nodule [43,44]. Nodule enhancement of less than 15 H is strongly predictive of a benign lesion whereas enhancement of greater than 20 H typically indicates malignancy with a sensitivity of 98%, specificity of 73%, and accuracy of 85% [43].

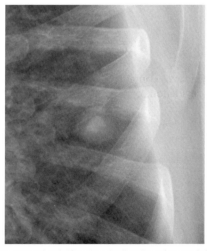

Fig. 3. Left lung nodule with dense central calcification indicating the nodule is a granuloma.

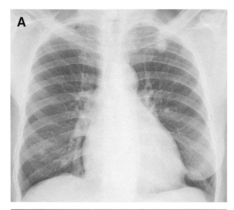

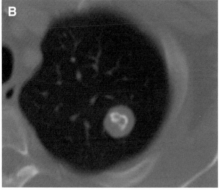

Fig. 4. (*A*) Left upper lobe nodule with "popcorn" calcification consistent with a hamartoma. (*B*) CT showing central calcifications with a "popcorn" appearance.

Attenuation

There are four basic tissue attenuations that can be recognized on plain radiograph or CT. These include: soft tissue density, calcified, fat containing on plain radiograph or CT, and ground glass on CT.

CT can characterize nodules as being nonsolid, partly solid, or solid. Approximately 34% of non-solid nodules are due to malignancy (Fig. 6) [45]. In a study by Suzuki and colleagues [46], 68% of ground glass lesions were bronchoalveolar cancers. Nonsolid lesions can be seen in benign conditions such as inflammatory disease and may even contain premalignant lesions such as atypical adenomatous hyperplasia or bronchoalveolar hyperplasia [47]. In a study by Henschke and colleagues [45], 63% of semisolid nodules (Fig. 7) were shown to be malignant compared with only 7% of solid nodules (Fig. 8). The risk of malignancy of a partly solid lesion increases with increasing size of the lesion and also if the solid component is centrally located [45,48].

Lipoid pneumonia can mimic a focal soft tissue mass, however, the demonstration of fat density on CT can confirm the diagnosis associated with

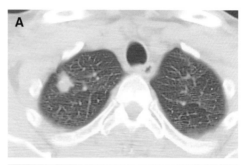

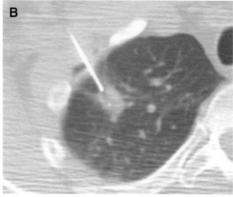

Fig. 5. (*A*) Right upper lobe nodule with eccentric calcification. (*B*) Fine needle aspiration biopsy yielding adenocarcinoma.

the use of mineral oil laxatives. Fat demonstrated within a nodule on CT is virtually diagnostic of a hamartoma (Fig. 9) [40]. On CT, approximately 60% of hamartomas contain fat with a measurement of −40 H to −120 H [40]. Metastasis from liposarcoma or renal cell carcinoma may occasionally contain fat [49].

Morphology

Certain lesions have a characteristic appearance on CT that allows a diagnosis to be determined based on imaging alone. These specific diagnoses include: arteriovenous fistula, rounded atelectasis, focal consolidation, pleural plaque, fungus ball, and mucus

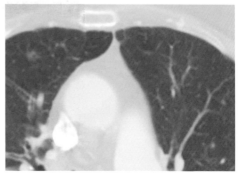

Fig. 6. Small right lung nonsolid nodule.

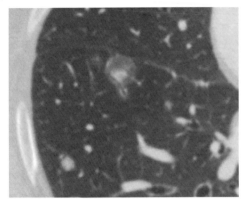

Fig. 7. Semisolid right lung nodule with an air bronchogram; fine needle biopsy yielding adenocarcinoma.

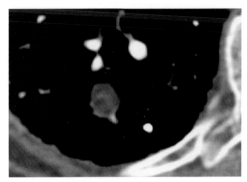

Fig. 9. CT scan of nodule demonstrates fat within the nodule indicating the nodule is a hamartoma.

plug. Thromboembolic disease with pulmonary infarction is suggested based on imaging appearance, but no specific defining imaging feature exists that confirms the diagnosis.

Arteriovenous fistulas often have a typical appearance on plain radiograph and CT, which includes a single, rounded, or serpiginous subpleural nodule with two feeding vessels, one arterial and one venous. If the diagnosis is suspected based on the plain film, the CT is usually obtained to confirm the diagnosis and also to evaluate for other arteriovenous fistulas, which are usually present in 35% of patients [37]. Although the diagnosis can usually be confirmed on CT without the use of intravenous contrast, contrast may be given to confirm the vascular nature of the lesion.

Rounded atelectasis is always associated with pleural disease. In fact, the following findings must be present to make a diagnosis of rounded atelectasis: ipsilateral pleural disease, extensive pleural contact, "comet-tail sign," and volume loss in the affected lobe. Even though the diagnosis may be made based on the appearance on a plain

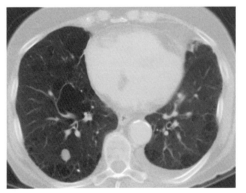

Fig. 8. Solid right lung nodule in a patient who has squamous cell carcinoma of the throat; fine needle biopsy shows changes consistent with a granuloma.

radiograph, it is much more specific when diagnosed with CT.

Fungus ball (aspergilloma) usually presents as a mass within a cavity. Air is usually seen that outlines the mass and is termed the "air crescent sign." When the lesion is imaged with the patient in various positions, there is movement of the mass within the cavity.

The diagnosis of mucus plug is made when there is a branching or tubular opacity noted in association with bronchial abnormalities. CT is much more accurate in making the diagnosis compared with plain radiography [37].

Although a radiograph may seem "normal" in thromboembolic disease, several underlying imaging abnormalities may be present. The nodular densities often seen are usually secondary to pulmonary infarction. Hampton's hump is defined by an opacity that is secondary to pulmonary hemorrhage into the secondary pulmonary lobules. Westermark's sign, a sign of oligemia, within the lung parenchyma is an uncommon finding. Bloody effusions indicate pulmonary infarction secondary to thromboemoblic disease [37]. Cavitation in an area of pulmonary infarction is usually secondary to infection. Rarely, a noninfected area of pulmonary infarction can undergo cavitation, which is a manifestation of pulmonary gangrene. Up to 15% of lung cancers cavitate, but most are greater than 3 cm in diameter [50].

Margin

Margin classifications include smooth, lobulated, irregular, and spiculated. Although a smooth and well-defined margin is suggestive of a benign diagnosis, as many as 21% of malignant lesions have well-defined margins (Fig. 10) [17]. Lobulated contours indicate uneven growth, which usually suggests a malignant etiology; however, up to 25% of benign lesions may have a lobulated contour (Fig. 11) [32,34]. Hamartomas are a prime example

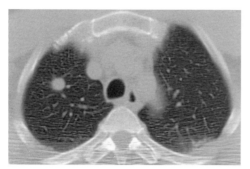

Fig. 10. Smoothly marginated RUL nodule proved to be a granuloma on fine needle biopsy evaluation.

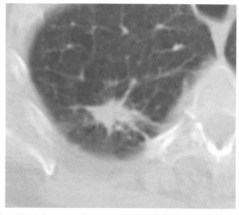

Fig. 12. Adenocarcinoma of the right upper lobe appearing as a spiculated nodule.

of benign lesions with a frequently lobulated contour.

A recent study demonstrated that all nodules with a halo margin, 97% with a densely spiculated margin (Fig. 12), 93% with a ragged margin, and 82% with a lobulated margin were malignant [51]. Irregular margins can be seen in some benign etiologies such as granulomatous disease, lipoid pneumonia, organizing pneumonia, and progressive massive fibrosis [18,52].

The contour with the highest predictive value for malignancy is an irregular or spiculated margin combined with distortion of the adjacent vessels (sunburst or corona radiata appearance) [18,32,34, 53,54]. A spiculated nodule has a positive predictive value of being malignant of approximately 90% [32].

Cavitation

Bubblelike lucencies or air bronchograms within a nodule are more often seen in malignant nodules

[34,55]. Air bronchograms are noted in up to 65% of adenocarcinomas but only 5% of benign SPNs (Fig. 13). Demonstration of a bronchus in a nodule with subsequent tapering and obstruction, abrupt obstruction of a bronchus by a nodule, and displacement of an airway around the periphery of a nodule with the airway intact are common in malignant nodules. The positive predictive values were 89%, 100%, and 93%, respectively. When bronchi course around the periphery of a nodule and the airway is compressed, the nodule is more likely benign with a 90% positive predictive value [56]. "Pseudocaviations," air-filled cystic regions, are common in adenocarcinomas and bronchioloalveolar carcinomas [37].

Cavitation is more common in malignant compared with benign nodules. Focal benign lesions such as pneumonia, however, can cavitate. The thickness of the wall is often evaluated to help determine the likelihood of benign versus malignant lesions. The thicker the wall, the more likely

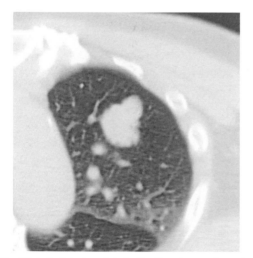

Fig. 11. Lobulated nodule in the lingula proving adenocarcinoma with fine needle biopsy.

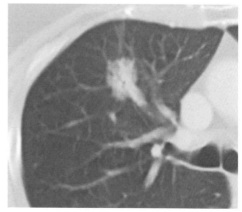

Fig. 13. Bronchoalveolar carcinoma appearing as a semi-solid nodule with air bronchograms.

the lesion is malignant (Fig. 14). In fact, it has been shown that all nodules with a wall thickness of 1 mm or less were benign and 84% of lesions with a wall thickness of 16 mm or more were malignant [57]. In the 5 mm to 15 mm range, 73% were benign. The internal margins of the walls of the cavity may also be helpful, because benign lesions tend to have smooth internal walls, whereas malignant lesions tend to have nodularity [5]. There is significant overlap in characteristics, however, preventing this feature from being used solely to determine a nodule as benign or malignant.

Growth rate

Traditionally, growth rates have been determined by evaluating changes in diameter of the nodule. However, with the advent of multidetector CT scanners and the development of software package on the associated CT workstations, it is much more accurate to use volumetric measurements. For example, a nodule that has doubled in volume will have only increased from 5 mm to 6.25 mm in diameter. This small change in diameter cannot be reliably detected on imaging. Typically, if a nodule doubles in volume in less than 1 month or more than 16 months, it is of benign etiology [37]. The doubling time for most malignant nodules is between 30 and 400 days. However, there is overlap in the growth rates of benign and malignant nodules making this a predictor and not an absolute indicator of benign or malignant etiology.

There is a generally accepted principal in the radiology community, which has been recently re-evaluated [58], that states if a nodule is stable and shows no growth over a 2-year period, then it is benign and does not require resection (Fig. 15). However, the positive predictive value for a benign disease in this situation is only 65% [6]. Even

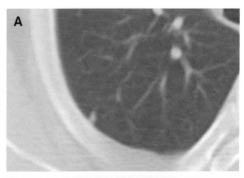

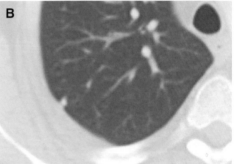

Fig. 15. (A) Small RLL nodule seen on initial CT scan. (B) Scan obtained two years latter shows no change in the size of the nodule and an increase in density due to the development of calcification. This indicates that the lesion is benign and most likely a granuloma.

though growth does not prove a nodule to be malignant, the likelihood that a growing nodule is malignant is much greater than that of a benign nodule (Fig. 16). This is one of the main reasons why prior radiographic examinations should always be obtained when evaluating a pulmonary nodule. The presence and stability of the nodule on a previous examination can prevent further workup—including biopsies or surgery—and can also prevent further radiographic evaluation, thus preventing unnecessary radiation exposure. If no prior examinations are available, further evaluation decisions will need to be made based on patient age, history, and radiographic appearance on the current examination.

Adjacent inflammatory changes, atelectasis, or scar may be accidentally included in the measurement of a nodule, which can be misleading because the lesion appears larger than it actually is. A nodule can then appear to grow if these adjacent changes have developed since the prior examination. More importantly, if the adjacent changes resolve between examinations, the nodule may appear to have decreased in size even though the underlying nodule is actually stable or even increased.

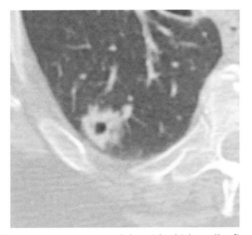

Fig. 14. RLL cavitary nodule with thick walls; fine needle biopsy diagnosed adenocarcinoma.

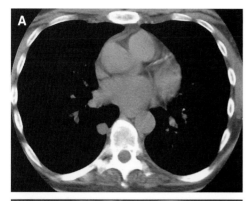

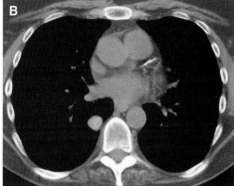

Fig. 16. (*A*) Right lower lobe non-calcified nodule, which on FNA was a granuloma. (*B*) Two years later the nodule is slightly larger. Density measurements show an increase in density due to the development of calcification within the nodule.

Bayesian analysis

Bayesian analysis can be helpful in the evaluation of indeterminate nodules. It uses likelihood ratios of numerous radiologic findings and clinical features to estimate the probability of malignancy in an SPN [32,59]. The mathematics is beyond the scope of this article. However, the application of this analysis is equivalent to or slightly superior to the evaluation of an SPN by an experienced radiologist in the risk stratification of benign and malignant nodules [32]. Clinical factors such as age and smoking history are included. Three clinical (age, smoking history, and previous malignancy) and three radiographic (diameter, spiculation, and upper lobe location) factors have been shown to be independent predictors of malignancy [60]. The probability for a particular patient can be calculated at the following Web site: http://www.chestx-ray.com/SPN/SPNProb.html.

Follow-up

Until recently, no guidelines for following an incidental pulmonary nodule discovered on routine CT scans were based on size criteria. The previous guidelines were written based on finding nodules on plain radiographs, which in general are larger than those found currently with multidetector CT scanners. Many incidental nodules are discovered during routine chest CT examinations measuring as small as 1 mm to 2 mm. These nodules are also frequently found in patients under the age of 35, in whom primary lung cancer is very rare (<1% of all cases). The Fleischner Society recently evaluated the available literature involving incidentally discovered pulmonary nodules and published a guideline of recommendations.

The primary scientific data supporting the follow-up of nodules are based on multiple publications relating to the various lung cancer screening trials currently being conducted. The one important conclusion was that nodules less than 5 mm in diameter have a very low likelihood (<1%) of being malignant in a patient without known malignancy [61–63]. In addition, the data from the Mayo Clinic CT Screening Trial demonstrated the likelihood of malignancy was 0.2% for nodules 3 mm or smaller, 0.9% for nodules 4 mm to 7 mm in diameter, 18% for 8 mm to 20 mm nodules, and 50% for those larger than 2 cm [64]. Therefore, based on this data, the Fleischner Society has made recommendations for following incidental nodules.

First, the patients are separated based on age into those younger or older than 35 years. Next, those older than 35 years are separated into a low- and high-risk population. Follow-up is then based on size criteria with these two different groups. The nodule size categories are: 4 mm or less, 4 mm to 6 mm, 6 mm to 8 mm, and greater than 8 mm in diameter. The recommendation range is from no follow-up needed in the case of a 4-mm or smaller nodule in a low-risk patient to 3-, 9-, and 24-month follow-up CT or consideration of dynamic contrast enhanced CT, PET, or biopsy in any patient with a nodule greater than 8 mm [64].

In general there has been a recommendation to follow a nodule for 2 years and if it has not changed in size, to suggest it is most likely benign. However, the one exception would be in a situation where the nodule is nonsolid (ground-glass) in appearance. This situation may require further follow-up, because nonsolid lesions have a greater likelihood of being malignant than solid lesions, and these can be relatively indolent [46,65].

There is no uniform recommendation for the management of indeterminate pulmonary nodules. For high or intermediate likelihood of malignancy, a reasonable approach is more aggressive intervention with needle biopsy or surgery. For those with a low likelihood of malignancy, it is reasonable to have the patient undergo close observation and follow-up with imaging. If new nodules develop during the time of observation, the risk of malignancy increases and more aggressive intervention seems reasonable.

Tissue diagnosis

Even if the CT is unable to assist in the definitive diagnosis of a benign versus malignant SPN, it can provide useful information for determining the etiology of the lesion, which often includes some form of tissue sampling. This can occur in various ways including percutaneous needle biopsy, bronchoscopy, mediastinoscopy, video-assisted thoracospoy, or thoracotomy. CT can help determine the best method with the highest chance of success based on the location and size of the nodule. Additional complicating factors such as emphysema can also be evaluated further. If it is determined not to obtain tissue, then CT can be a good modality for following the nodule for growth assessment or for morphologic changes that would suggest a malignant etiology.

Transthoracic needle biopsy has a 95% to 100% sensitivity rate for diagnosing malignant nodules in those less than 10 mm to 15 mm in diameter (Fig. 17) [66–68]. Needle aspiration biopsy has

a significant false-negative rate of approximately 10% in diagnosing carcinomas [37]. Although specific benign diagnoses are sometimes difficult, needle biopsy has a reported benign diagnosis in 91% of patients [69]. Complications include pneumothorax in 5% to 30% of patients [66,70,71]. Approximately 15% of patients who have pneumothorax require chest tube placement [66,71]. Minor hemoptysis or pulmonary hemorrhage occurs in approximately 3% of patients [72]. Air embolism is a rare complication of needle biopsy, which may present as stroke, transient ischemic attack, seizure, or cardiopulmonary collapse. Fine needle aspiration (FNA) contraindications include: inability of patient to cooperate, bleeding diathesis, previous pneumonectomy, severe emphysema, severe hypoxemia, or pulmonary artery hypertension. Core biopsies can be reserved for cases where FNA fails to provide a specific tissue diagnosis. If a malignant or specific benign diagnosis is not obtained with needle biopsy then further evaluation is required.

Bronchoscopy is more accurate in diagnosing central masses, which have an endobronchial component compared with needle biopsy, which is best suited for sampling peripheral lesions.

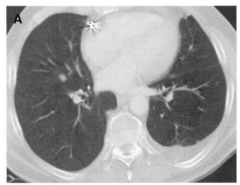

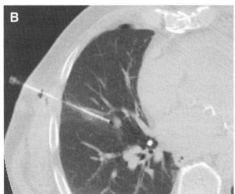

Fig. 17. (*A*) Smoothly marginated non-calcified nodule in the right middle lobe. (*B*) FNA of the nodule demonstrate adenocarcinoma.

References

[1] Erasmus JJ, Connolly JE, McAdams HP, et al. Solitary pulmonary nodules: part I. Morphologic evaluation for differentiation of benign and malignant lesions. Radiographics 2000;20(1): 43–58.

[2] Swensen SJ, Silverstein MD, Edell ES, et al. Solitary pulmonary nodules: clinical prediction model versus physicians. Mayo Clin Proc 1999; 74(4):319–29.

[3] Bateson EM. An analysis of 155 solitary lung lesions illustrating the differential diagnosis of mixed tumours of the lung. Clin Radiol 1965; 16:51–65.

[4] Murthy SC, Rice TW. The solitary pulmonary nodule: a primer on differential diagnosis. Semin Thorac Cardiovasc Surg 2002;14(3):239–49.

[5] Hartman TE. Radiologic evaluation of the solitary pulmonary nodule. Radiol Clin North Am 2005;43(3):459–65.

[6] Erasmus JJ, McAdams HP, Connolly JE. Solitary pulmonary nodules: part II. Evaluation of the indeterminate nodule. Radiographics 2000;20(1): 59–66.

[7] Quint LE, Park CH, Iannettoni MD. Solitary pulmonary nodules in patients with extrapulmonary neoplasms. Radiology 2000;217(1):257–61.

[8] Kundel HL. Predictive value and threshold detectability of lung tumors. Radiology 1981; 139(1):25–9.

[9] Niklason LT, Hickey NM, Chakraborty DP, et al. Simulated pulmonary nodules: detection with

dual-energy digital versus conventional radiography. Radiology 1986;160(3):589–93.

[10] Muhm JR, Miller WE, Fontana RS, et al. Lung cancer detected during a screening program using four-month chest radiographs. Radiology 1983;148(3):609–15.

[11] Austin JH, Romney BM, Goldsmith LS. Missed bronchogenic carcinoma: radiographic findings in 27 patients with a potentially resectable lesion evident in retrospect. Radiology 1992;182(1):115–22.

[12] Shah PK, Austin JH, White CS, et al. Missed non-small cell lung cancer: radiographic findings of potentially resectable lesions evident only in retrospect. Radiology 2003;226(1):235–41.

[13] Huston J 3rd, Muhm JR. Solitary pulmonary nodules: evaluation with a CT reference phantom. Radiology 1989;170(3 Pt 1):653–6.

[14] Proto AV, Thomas SR. Pulmonary nodules studied by computed tomography. Radiology 1985;156(1):149–53.

[15] Siegelman SS, Khouri NF, Leo FP, et al. Solitary pulmonary nodules: CT assessment. Radiology 1986;160(2):307–12.

[16] Khouri NF, Meziane MA, Zerhouni EA, et al. The solitary pulmonary nodule. Assessment, diagnosis, and management. Chest 1987;91(1):128–33.

[17] Siegelman SS, Zerhouni EA, Leo FP, et al. CT of the solitary pulmonary nodule. AJR Am J Roentgenol 1980;135(1):1–13.

[18] Zerhouni EA, Stitik FP, Siegelman SS, et al. CT of the pulmonary nodule: a cooperative study. Radiology 1986;160(2):319–27.

[19] Im JG, Gamsu G, Gordon D, et al. CT densitometry of pulmonary nodules in a frozen human thorax. AJR Am J Roentgenol 1988;150(1):61–6.

[20] Swensen SJ, Jett JR, Sloan JA, et al. Screening for lung cancer with low-dose spiral computed tomography. Am J Respir Crit Care Med 2002;165(4):508–13.

[21] Ko JP, Rusinek H, Naidich DP, et al. Wavelet compression of low-dose chest CT data: effect on lung nodule detection. Radiology 2003;228(1):70–5.

[22] Coakley FV, Cohen MD, Johnson MS, et al. Maximum intensity projection images in the detection of simulated pulmonary nodules by spiral CT. Br J Radiol 1998;71(842):135–40.

[23] Gruden JF, Ouanounou S, Tigges S, et al. Incremental benefit of maximum-intensity-projection images on observer detection of small pulmonary nodules revealed by multidetector CT. AJR Am J Roentgenol 2002;179(1):149–57.

[24] Rusinek H, Naidich DP, McGuinness G, et al. Pulmonary nodule detection: low-dose versus conventional CT. Radiology 1998;209(1):243–9.

[25] Tillich M, Kammerhuber F, Reittner P, et al. Detection of pulmonary nodules with helical CT: comparison of cine and film-based viewing. AJR Am J Roentgenol 1997;169(6):1611–4.

[26] Swensen SJ, Viggiano RW, Midthun DE, et al. Lung nodule enhancement at CT: multicenter study. Radiology 2000;214(1):73–80.

[27] Winer-Muram HT, Jennings SG, Tarver RD, et al. Volumetric growth rate of stage I lung cancer prior to treatment: serial CT scanning. Radiology 2002;223(3):798–805.

[28] Lee HJ, Im JG, Ahn JM, et al. Lung cancer in patients with idiopathic pulmonary fibrosis: CT findings. J Comput Assist Tomogr 1996;20(6):979–82.

[29] Quinn D, Gianlupi A, Broste S. The changing radiographic presentation of bronchogenic carcinoma with reference to cell types. Chest 1996;110(6):1474–9.

[30] Bower SL, Choplin RH, Muss HB. Multiple primary bronchogenic carcinomas of the lung. AJR Am J Roentgenol 1983;140(2):253–8.

[31] Stark P. Multiple independent bronchogenic carcinomas. Radiology 1982;145(3):599–601.

[32] Gurney JW. Determining the likelihood of malignancy in solitary pulmonary nodules with Bayesian analysis. Part I. Theory. Radiology 1993;186(2):405–13.

[33] Higgins GA, Shields TW, Keehn RJ. The solitary pulmonary nodule. Ten-year follow-up of veterans administration-armed forces cooperative study. Arch Surg 1975;110(5):570–5.

[34] Zwirewich CV, Vedal S, Miller RR, et al. Solitary pulmonary nodule: high-resolution CT and radiologic-pathologic correlation. Radiology 1991;179(2):469–76.

[35] Viggiano RW, Swensen SJ, Rosenow EC 3rd. Evaluation and management of solitary and multiple pulmonary nodules. Clin Chest Med 1992;13(1):83–95.

[36] Berger WG, Erly WK, Krupinski EA, et al. The solitary pulmonary nodule on chest radiography: can we really tell if the nodule is calcified? AJR Am J Roentgenol 2001;176(1):201–4.

[37] Freundlich IM, Bragg DG. A radiologic approach to diseases of the chest. 2nd ed. Baltimore (MD): Williams & Wilkins; 1997.

[38] Ledor K, Fish B, Chaise L, Ledor S. CT diagnosis of pulmonary hamartomas. J Comput Tomogr 1981;5(4):343–4.

[39] Oldham HN Jr, Young WG Jr, Sealy WC. Hamartoma of the lung. J Thorac Cardiovasc Surg 1967;53(5):735–42.

[40] Siegelman SS, Khouri NF, Scott WW Jr, et al. Pulmonary hamartoma: CT findings. Radiology 1986;160(2):313–7.

[41] Mahoney MC, Shipley RT, Corcoran HL, et al. CT demonstration of calcification in carcinoma of the lung. AJR Am J Roentgenol 1990;154(2):255–8.

[42] Swensen SJ, Brown LR, Colby TV, et al. Pulmonary nodules: CT evaluation of enhancement with iodinated contrast material. Radiology 1995;194(2):393–8.

[43] Swensen SJ, Brown LR, Colby TV, et al. Lung nodule enhancement at CT: prospective findings. Radiology 1996;201(2):447–55.

[44] Yamashita K, Matsunobe S, Tsuda T, et al. Solitary pulmonary nodule: preliminary study of

evaluation with incremental dynamic CT. Radiology 1995;194(2):399–405.

[45] Henschke CI, Yankelevitz DF, Mirtcheva R, et al. CT screening for lung cancer: frequency and significance of part-solid and nonsolid nodules. AJR Am J Roentgenol 2002;178(5):1053–7.

[46] Suzuki K, Asamura H, Kusumoto M, et al. "Early" peripheral lung cancer: prognostic significance of ground glass opacity on thin-section computed tomographic scan. Ann Thorac Surg 2002;74(5):1635–9.

[47] Vazquez M, Flieder D, Travis W, et al. Early lung cancer action project pathology protocol. Lung Cancer 2003;39(2):231–2.

[48] Li F, Sone S, Abe H, et al. Malignant versus benign nodules at CT screening for lung cancer: comparison of thin-section CT findings. Radiology 2004;233(3):793–8.

[49] Muram TM, Aisen A. Fatty metastatic lesions in 2 patients with renal clear-cell carcinoma. J Comput Assist Tomogr 2003;27(6):869–70.

[50] Chaudhuri MR. Primary pulmonary cavitating carcinomas. Thorax 1973;28(3):354–66.

[51] Furuya K, Murayama S, Soeda H, et al. New classification of small pulmonary nodules by margin characteristics on high-resolution CT. Acta Radiol 1999;40(5):496–504.

[52] Huston J 3rd, Muhm JR. Solitary pulmonary opacities: plain tomography. Radiology 1987;163(2):481–5.

[53] Sider L. Radiographic manifestations of primary bronchogenic carcinoma. Radiol Clin North Am 1990;28(3):583–97.

[54] Theros EG. 1976 Caldwell lecture: varying manifestation of peripheral pulmonary neoplasms: a radiologic-pathologic correlative study. AJR Am J Roentgenol 1977;128(6):893–914.

[55] Kuriyama K, Tateishi R, Doi O, et al. Prevalence of air bronchograms in small peripheral carcinomas of the lung on thin-section CT: comparison with benign tumors. AJR Am J Roentgenol 1991;156(5):921–4.

[56] Qiang JW, Zhou KR, Lu G, et al. The relationship between solitary pulmonary nodules and bronchi: multi-slice CT-pathological correlation. Clin Radiol 2004;59(12):1121–7.

[57] Woodring JH, Fried AM. Significance of wall thickness in solitary cavities of the lung: a follow-up study. AJR Am J Roentgenol 1983;140(3):473–4.

[58] Yankelevitz DF, Henschke CI. Does 2-year stability imply that pulmonary nodules are benign? AJR Am J Roentgenol 1997;168(2):325–8.

[59] Black WC, Armstrong P. Communicating the significance of radiologic test results: the likelihood ratio. AJR Am J Roentgenol 1986;147(6):1313–8.

[60] Swensen SJ, Silverstein MD, Ilstrup DM, et al. The probability of malignancy in solitary pulmonary nodules. Application to small radiologically indeterminate nodules. Arch Intern Med 1997; 157(8):849–55.

[61] Henschke CI, McCauley DI, Yankelevitz DF, et al. Early Lung Cancer Action Project: overall design and findings from baseline screening. Lancet 1999;354(9173):99–105.

[62] Henschke CI, Yankelevitz DF, Naidich DP, et al. CT screening for lung cancer: suspiciousness of nodules according to size on baseline scans. Radiology 2004;231(1):164–8.

[63] Swensen SJ, Jett JR, Hartman TE, et al. Lung cancer screening with CT: Mayo Clinic experience. Radiology 2003;226(3):756–61.

[64] MacMahon H, Austin JH, Gamsu G, et al. Guidelines for management of small pulmonary nodules detected on CT scans: a statement from the Fleischner Society. Radiology 2005;237(2): 395–400.

[65] Hasegawa M, Sone S, Takashima S, et al. Growth rate of small lung cancers detected on mass CT screening. Br J Radiol 2000;73(876):1252–9.

[66] Klein JS, Zarka MA. Transthoracic needle biopsy: an overview. J Thorac Imaging 1997;12(4): 232–49.

[67] Li H, Boiselle PM, Shepard JO, et al. Diagnostic accuracy and safety of CT-guided percutaneous needle aspiration biopsy of the lung: comparison of small and large pulmonary nodules. AJR Am J Roentgenol 1996;167(1):105–9.

[68] Westcott JL, Rao N, Colley DP. Transthoracic needle biopsy of small pulmonary nodules. Radiology 1997;202(1):97–103.

[69] Klein JS, Salomon G, Stewart EA. Transthoracic needle biopsy with a coaxially placed 20-gauge automated cutting needle: results in 122 patients. Radiology 1996;198(3):715–20.

[70] Miller JA, Pramanik BK, Lavenhar MA. Predicting the rates of success and complications of computed tomography-guided percutaneous core-needle biopsies of the thorax from the findings of the preprocedure chest computed tomography scan. J Thorac Imaging 1998;13(1):7–13.

[71] Moore EH. Needle-aspiration lung biopsy: a comprehensive approach to complication reduction. J Thorac Imaging 1997;12(4):259–71.

[72] Arslan S, Yilmaz A, Bayramgurler B, et al. CT-guided transthoracic fine needle aspiration of pulmonary lesions: accuracy and complications in 294 patients. Med Sci Monit 2002;8(7): CR493–7.

ELSEVIER
SAUNDERS

POSITRON
EMISSION
TOMOGRAPHY

PET Clin 1 (2006) 301–316

Staging of Lung Cancer

Jokke Wynants, MD[a], Sigrid Stroobants, MD, PhD[b],
Christophe Dooms, MD[a], Johan Vansteenkiste, MD, PhD[a],*

- The staging system of lung cancer
- Baseline staging: T factor
  Evaluation of pleural disease
- Baseline staging: N factor
- Baseline staging: M factor
- Baseline staging: consequences of PET in the work-up of non-small cell lung cancer

Guidance of invasive procedures
Impact on overall stage and management
- Small cell lung cancer
- Restaging after induction therapy
- Pitfalls in staging lung cancer with PET
  False-negative findings
  False-positive findings
- References

Lung cancer is the most common cause of cancer-related death in the Western world, with approximately 1.2 million new cases per year worldwide. Imaging techniques play a vital role in the diagnosis, staging, and follow-up of patients who have lung cancer. For this purpose, PET has become an important adjunct to conventional imaging techniques such as chest radiography, CT, ultrasonography, and MR imaging [1]. The ability of PET to differentiate the metabolic properties of tissues allows more accurate assessment of undetermined lung lesions, mediastinal lymph nodes (LNs), or extrathoracic abnormalities, tumor response after induction treatment, and detection of disease recurrence [2].

The standard tracer in lung cancer PET imaging is the glucose analogue ^{18}F-fluoro-2-deoxy-D-glucose (FDG). FDG allows excellent discrimination between normal tissues and tissues with enhanced glucose metabolism, but false-positive uptake of FDG in inflammatory tissues is one of its major limitations. Therefore, tracers with an equally high sensitivity but a better specificity are the focus of ongoing research. Other tracers such as

^{11}C-methionine (a marker of protein metabolism), ^{11}C-choline (a marker of the cell membrane component phosphaditylcholine), and ^{18}F-fluorothymidine (a marker of cell proliferation) have been studied. The experience with these tracers is still limited. At this time they have not shown a clear advantage over FDG in clinical lung cancer imaging, and they are not discussed further in this article.

Most of the studies in lung cancer were performed with a full-ring (or "dedicated") PET camera, and they are the basis for the recommendations for the use of PET in clinical decisions. It is not clear, and is even doubtful, if the same recommendations apply to dual-head coincidence gamma camera imaging.

The staging system of lung cancer

For the past 2 decades, the international staging system for lung cancer has provided a common language for communication about patients. Accurate staging is essential to make estimates of prognosis

[a] Respiratory Oncology Unit (Pulmonology), Leuven Lung Cancer Group, University Hospital Gasthuisberg, Catholic University, Herestraat 49, B-3000, Leuven, Belgium
[b] PET Center (Nuclear Medicine), University Hospital Gasthuisberg, Catholic University, Herestraat 49, B-3000, Leuven, Belgium
* Corresponding author.
E-mail address: johan.vansteenkiste@uz.kuleuven.ac.be (J. Vansteenkiste).

doi:10.1016/j.cpet.2006.10.002

and to choose the best combination of treatment modalities such as surgery, radiotherapy, and chemotherapy in an attempt to improve survival.

The system defines the TNM category of each patient who has non–small cell lung cancer (NSCLC) (Table 1) [3]. The T factor describes the primary tumor by size and invasiveness, ranging from T1 (< 3 cm and entirely surrounded by lung tissue) to T4 (invading critical organs such as the aorta). The N factor describes the locoregional LN spread, either no metastatic nodes (N0), to intrapulmonary or hilar nodes only (N1), to ipsilateral mediastinal nodes (N2), or to contralateral mediastinal or supraclavicular nodes (N3). The M factor denotes absence (M0) or presence (M1) of distant metastasis.

A major step forward in the latest staging system has been the adoption of a unique system for N-factor staging. Previously, there were two mediastinal LN classifications, one by Naruke [4] and the other by the American Thoracic Society [5]. The map published in 1997 was recognized by the American Joint Committee on Cancer and the TNM Committee of the Union Internationale Contre le Cancer (Fig. 1) [6]. The three groups of mediastinal LNs are indicated by a single digit: superior (1–4), aortic (5 or 6), and inferior (7–9). Hilar (10) and intrapulmonary (11–13) LNs have a double digit. This map can be used to interpret imaging studies and to guide LN sampling procedures such as endoscopic needle aspirations or mediastinoscopy [7]. The pattern of LN spread;depends, in general, on the site of the primary tumor. Right upper- and middle-lobe tumors often spread to the right hilar and right superior mediastinal nodes, right lower-lobe tumors often spread to the right hilar and inferior mediastinal stations. Left upper-lobe tumors have a predilection for left hilar, aortic, and left paratracheal nodes; left lower-lobe tumors spread to the left hilar nodes and the inferior mediastinal nodes, with a high tendency to cross the midline.

Based on their TNM denominators, patients are grouped into stages with more-or-less homogeneous prognosis. The current system distinguishes seven stages of disease, each with a different outcome (see Table 1). For therapeutic considerations, stage I and stage ,II disease are often referred to as "early stage"; for these patients the standard of care is local treatment, preferably resection followed by adjuvant chemotherapy except for stage IA [8], or radical radiotherapy in case of poor cardiopulmonary function. Patients who have stage III disease have locally advanced disease, either IIIA (N2: LN spread in the ipsilateral mediastinal nodes only) or IIIB (N3: LN spread in the contralateral mediastinal or supraclavicular nodes). Except for patients who have IIIB stage based on T4 malignant pleural effusion, a combination of local and systemic treatment offers the best prospects for remission, or sometimes cure. In North America, this treatment often is concurrent chemoradiotherapy [9]. Many European centers treat patients who have stage IIIA disease with induction therapy followed by attempted

Table 1:	TNM staging of lung cancer			
Stage	Tumor	Node	Metastasis	Definition
IA	T1	N0	M0	T1 tumor: ≤3 cm, surrounded by lung or pleura; no tumor more proximal than lobe bronchus
IB	T2	N0	M0	T2 tumor: >3cm, involving main bronchus ≥2 cm distal to carina, invading pleura; atelectasis or pneumonitis extending to hilum but not entire lung
IIA	T1	N1	M0	N1: involvement of ipsilateral peribronchial or hilar nodes and intra, pulmonary nodes by direct extension
IIB	T2	N1	M0	
	T3	N0	M0	T3 tumor: invasion of chest wall, diaphragm. mediastinal pleura, pericardium, main bronchus <2 cm distal to carina; atelectasis or pneumonitis of entire lung
IIIA	T1	N2	M0	
	T2	N2	M0	
	T3	N1	M0	
	T3	N2	M0	N2: involvement ipsilateral mediastinal or subcarinal nodes
IIIB	Any T	N3	M0	N3: involvement of contralateral (lung) nodes or any supraclavicular node
IIIB	T4	Any N	M0	T4 tumor: invasion of mediastinum, heart, great vessels, trachea, esophagus, vertebral body, carina; separate tumor nodules; malignant pleural effusion
IV	Any T	Any N	M1	Distant metastasis

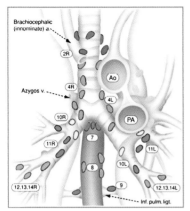

Superior Mediastinal Nodes

● **1** Highest Mediastinal

● **2** Upper Paratracheal

○ **3** Pre-vascular and Retrotracheal

○ **4** Lower Paratracheal
(including Azygos Nodes)

N_2 = single digit, ipsilateral
N_3 = single digit, contralateral or supraclavicular

Aortic Nodes

● **5** Subaortic (A-P window)

○ **6** Para-aortic (ascending
aorta or phrenic)

Inferior Mediastinal Nodes

○ **7** Subcarinal

○ **8** Paraesophageal
(below carina)

○ **9** Pulmonary Ligament

N₁ Nodes

○ **10** Hilar

● **11** Interlobar

○ **12** Lobar

○ **13** Segmental

○ **14** Subsegmental

Fig. 1. Lung cancer lymph node map according to Mountain and Dressler. Ao, aorta; L, left; N_2, single-digit, ipsilateral; N_3, single-digit, contralateral or supraclavicular; PA, pulmonary artery; R, right; 1, highest mediastinal node; 2, upper paratracheal nodes; 3, prevascular and retrotracheal nodes; 4, lower paratracheal nodes; 5, subaortic nodes (aortopulmonary window); 6, para-aortic nodes (ascending aorta or phrenic); 7, subcarinal nodes; 8, paraesophageal nodes (below carina); 9, pulmonary ligament; 10, hilar nodes; 11, interlobar nodes; 12, lobar nodes; 13, segmental nodes; 14, subsegmental nodes. (*Courtesy of* Clifton F. Mountain, MD, San Diego, CA, with permission. © Copyright 1996, Mountain and Dresler.)

complete resection [10–13]. Patients who have stage IV (advanced or metastatic) disease are no longer amenable to cure. Chemotherapy results in a moderate improvement of the median survival, subjective clinical benefit [14], or quality of life [15].

Baseline staging: T factor

In general, CT has gained a central role in lung cancer staging and now is appropriate for every treatable patient. MR imaging can be of additional benefit in some instances (eg, by showing superior sulcus extension or the relationship with the heart or large vessels) [16]. With its excellent anatomic detail, however, modern CT is the best choice to assess the T factor, that is, the relationship of the tumor to the fissures (which may determine the type of resection), to mediastinal structures, or to the pleura and chest wall. For the assessment of primary tumor extension, CT with its better spatial resolution remains the standard test. CT criteria for probable resectability in masses contiguous with the mediastinum are a contact with mediastinum of less than 3 cm, less than 90° contact with aorta, and preserved mediastinal fat layer between the mass and mediastinal structures. The reverse findings (ie, >3-cm

contact with mediastinum, > 90° contact with aorta, obliteration of the fat plane between mass and mediastinal structures) are not reliable signs of either invasion or nonresectability [17–19]. Consequently, CT often does not obviate surgical exploration, because it provides reliable signs of resectability but less reliable signs of nonresectability. The same is true for chest wall invasion, with the exception of the 100% positive predictive value of bony rib destruction with or without a soft tissue mass extending into the chest wall [16,20,21].

PET by itself does not add much to the assessment of local resectability, because its inferior spatial resolution does not provide more detail of the exact tumor extent or infiltration of neighboring structures. Recently, one prospective study of 40 patients reported that PET-CT fusion images provided more precise information for the evaluation of chest wall and mediastinal infiltration in some patients because of better differentiation between tumor and peritumoral inflammation or atelectasis [22]. A review of the experience at the Leuven Lung Cancer Group (LLCG) with fusion PET-CT, in comparison with CT alone, PET alone, and side-to-side correlated PET-CT, revealed a sensitivity for fusion PET-CT of 83%, a specificity of 84%, and an accuracy of 84%

[23]. These results were significantly better than for CT alone or PET alone, but there was no benefit in comparison with side-to-side correlated PET-CT.

Evaluation of pleural disease

The presence of pleural fluid in a patient who has lung cancer always should raise the possibility of pleural tumor spread, thereby changing the T factor from T1–T3 to T4 and thus changing staging to stage IIIB, no longer amenable to potentially radical therapy. Malignant pleural effusion should, however, be differentiated from nonmalignant fluid, which can be caused by atelectasis, pneumonia, or impairment of lymphatic drainage.

In a first retrospective report on 25 patients who had NSCLC and suspected malignant pleural effusions, PET was reported to have a sensitivity of 95% (21/22 patients) [24]. Because only three patients in this series had benign pleural disease, specificity could not be judged truly. In another study with a prevalence of malignant pleural involvement of about 50%, PET correctly detected the presence of malignant pleural involvement in 16 of 18 patients and excluded malignant pleural involvement in 16 of 17 patients (sensitivity 89%, specificity 94%, accuracy 91%) [25]. In a later study of pleural effusion in 92 patients, of whom 71% were deemed indeterminate on CT, PET had a sensitivity, specificity, and accuracy of 100%, 71%, and 80%, respectively, and PET/CT had a sensitivity, specificity, and accuracy of 100%, 76%, and 84%, respectively [26]. In this particular study, specificity and positive predictive value were lower, because of the larger number of benign pleural effusions.

The outcome of these studies thus varies according to the type of patients included and the prevalence of malignancy in the total number of effusions. PET thus can be useful in evaluating pleural disease in patients who have lung cancer but nonetheless should be interpreted with caution. Small or flat pleural deposits can indeed be missed on PET, probably because of their low tumor load or partial volume effects (Fig. 2) [27]. On the other hand, false-positive findings may occur in patients who have inflammatory pleural lesions. If the pleural staging determines the chances for radical treatment, pathologic verification with cytology or thoracoscopic biopsy should be sought.

Baseline staging: N factor

The N stage describes the presence and extent of locoregional LN invasion in NSCLC, and strongly determines the prognosis and the choice of treatment when distant metastases are absent. For patients who do not have positive LNs or who have only intrapulmonary or hilar ones, direct resection remains standard therapy. In case of positive ipsilateral mediastinal LNs (N2), induction treatment followed by surgery is a choice for resectable patients; others are treated with a combination of chemotherapy and radiotherapy [10,28]. Patients who have contralateral metastatic mediastinal LNs (N3 disease) generally are not candidates for surgery but receive nonsurgical combined modality treatment.

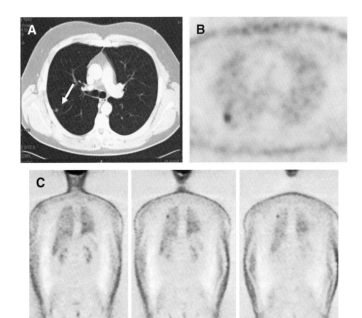

Fig. 2. (*A*) Detection of a small pulmonary nodule on a CT made for vague right-sided thoracic pain in a 41-year-old patient. (*B, C*) The lesion is FDG avid. There are no signs of lymph node or pleural disease and no explanation for thoracic pain. At thoracoscopy, diffuse superficial pleural metastases from a lung adenocarcinoma were present.

For years CT has been the standard noninvasive staging method for the mediastinum. Enlarged LNs (ie, > 10 mm in the short axis) were considered to be metastatic. Size is a relative criterion, however, because there can be infectious or inflammatory causes for LNs enlargement, and small nodes can contain metastatic deposits. The sensitivity and specificity of thoracic CT for detection of mediastinal LN spread were only 69% and 71%, respectively, in one large series [29]. In a review, the pooled sensitivity of CT was 57% (95% confidence interval [CI], 49%–66%) and the specificity was 82% (95% CI, 77%–86%) [30].

During the last years, several prospective studies yielded strong evidence that PET is significantly more accurate than thoracic CT for assessing the N factor in NSCLC. In a landmark LLCG study, PET proved significantly more accurate than CT in LN staging, and if CT and PET images were correlated, the negative predictive value of 95% proved to be slightly better than the one reported in mediastinoscopy series [31]. This superiority has been confirmed in five meta-analyses [30,32–35]. PET correctly identifies large benign nodes and also small malignant nodes because of the high contrast resolution of FDG-avid LN metastases on PET (Fig. 3). In a comparative study, the sensitivity, specificity, and accuracy of PET for detecting small (<1 cm in size) malignant LNs were 80%, 95%, and 92% respectively, and for LNs of 1 to 3 cm were 100%, 91%, and 95%, respectively [36].

The high negative predictive value is the true strength of PET. It creates the possibility of avoiding invasive staging if PET suggests the absence of LN disease. This negative predictive value is valid only when there is sufficient FDG uptake in the primary tumor and in the absence of a central tumor or important hilar LN disease that may obscure coexisting N2 disease [37]. If these rules of interpretation are observed, relevant LN disease rarely is missed. In some patients, LNs with small tumor deposits, ranging from 1 to 7.5 mm [38], may remain undetected because of the spatial resolution of the PET camera. In these patients, minimal N2 disease may be discovered at surgical exploration, but resection in these patients is rewarding [39,40].

The positive predictive value of PET is less optimal. Therefore, in case of positive LN findings on PET, tissue confirmation is mandatory to avoid radical surgery in node-free patients based on false-positive findings (eg, caused by granulomatous or other inflammatory conditions).

The available studies indicate that visual correlation with CT images is the minimal standard to optimize PET interpretation [41–43]. Fusion PET-CT images are one step further, with the obvious advantage of decreasing the learning curve needed to optimize the visual correlation (Fig. 4). The advantages of this approach are discussed elsewhere in this issue.

Baseline staging: M factor

The observation of metastases in patients who have NSCLC implies that a patient can no longer be cured. Forty percent of the patients who have NSCLC have distant metastases at presentation, most commonly in the adrenal glands, bones, liver, or brain [44]. The current standard noninvasive staging tests (including ultrasound, CT, MR imaging, and bone scintigraphy) are far from perfect. A systemic relapse develops in up to 20% of surgically treated patients within 3 to 24 months after complete surgical resection. The explanation of the high false-negative rate of conventional imaging

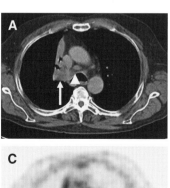
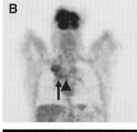
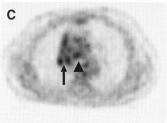
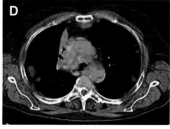

Fig. 3. (*A*) CT scan of a patient who has a centrally located right upper lobe tumor (*arrow*) and a small lymph node in the right paratracheal space (*arrowhead*). (*B, C*) FDG uptake in the tumor, hilar (*arrow*), and right mediastinal nodes (*arrowhead*). (*D*) Fusion images clearly suggest mediastinal lymph node spread, which was confirmed at cervical mediastinoscopy.

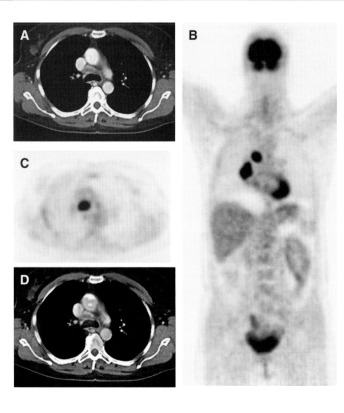

Fig. 4. (A) CT of a patient who has a centrally located right lung tumor (not shown) and adenopathy. (B, C) On PET images, adenopathy can be either right hilar, right mediastinal, or both. (D) Fusion images confirm that the lymph node metastasis has a right paratracheal location (4R in Fig. 1).

probably lies in the presence of micrometastatic spread at the time of diagnosis of biologically more aggressive tumors [45].

PET offers a double additional value in the evaluation of distant metastases in patients who have potentially operable NSCLC. On the one hand, there is the detection of unexpected metastatic spread, which occurs in 5% to 29% of patients who have negative conventional imaging (Fig. 5) [46–59]. This broad range is explained by several factors. First is the variability in the extent or rigor of the pre-PET extrathoracic conventional imaging. Second, in some studies the equivocal lesions are regarded as unexpected metastases if PET confirms malignancy in these lesions [47,48], but this is not the case in most other studies. Finally, the chance of detecting metastases on PET varies with the population in the study, being found in 7% of the patients who have pre-PET stage I disease, in 18% of patients who have stage II disease, and in up to 24% of patients who have stage III disease [53]. Focal unexpected FDG-PET uptake in sites unlikely to be metastatic for NSCLC also may reveal a second primary tumor in some patients (eg, colorectal or breast cancer) (Fig. 6).

On the other hand, lesions that are equivocal on conventional imaging can be assessed further by PET. Because of the very high sensitivity of PET in the detection of adrenal metastases, a negative PET image of an equivocal adrenal lesion on CT

usually indicates a nonmetastatic cause [60–62]. This indication is important, because up to 10% of patients who have NSCLC have an adrenal mass at the time of staging, and about one half to two thirds of these lesions are benign [63,64]. Caution is required in lesions smaller than 1 cm. Specificity of PET for adrenal metastases is high (between 80% and 100%), but some false-positive lesions have been described.

The evaluation of bone metastases in NSCLC by PET has a sensitivity at least equal to that of Technetium-99m bone scan (about 90%) but has a better specificity [65–69], 98% versus 61% in one study [65]. Caution, however, is required with distal lesions (eg, below the knee) that fall outside the field of view of a standard "whole-body" PET acquisition and with osteoblastic lesions, which are more readily seen on Technetium-99m bone scan, as demonstrated in a study of patients who had breast cancer [70]. Because most bone lesions in NSCLC are in the central skeleton, and nearly all are osteolytic, PET scan usually replaces bone scan, except in specific clinical indications.

The standard method for the detection of liver metastases is ultrasonography or CT. There are no specific series on the use of PET in patients who have liver metastases from NSCLC. Some general series on staging NSCLC suggest that PET is more accurate than CT [47,50]. Other series on different types of tumors have reported a nonsignificant

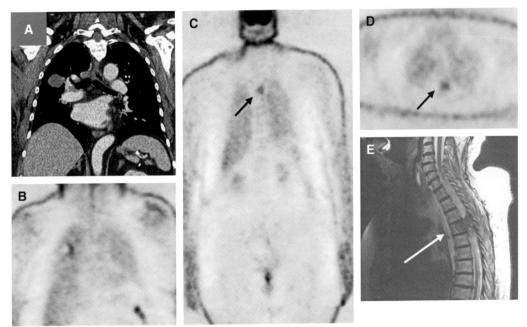

Fig. 5. (*A*, *B*) The patient has large cell lung cancer in the right upper lobe. (*C*, *D*) There is a suspected bone lesion in the thoracic spine (*arrow*). (*E*) Bone CT was equivocal, but MR imaging of the spine confirmed bone and soft tissue metastasis (*arrow*).

difference in sensitivity (93% versus 97%), specificity (75% versus 88%), and accuracy (85% versus 92%) for CT and PET, respectively, in the detection of liver involvement [71,72]. Thus, ultrasonography and CT remain the standard imaging techniques for the liver. Additional diagnostic information is provided by PET combined with CT, namely in the differentiation of hepatic lesions that are indeterminate on conventional imaging [71].

FDG-PET is not sensitive enough to exclude brain metastases, because of the high glucose uptake of normal surrounding brain tissue. MR imaging (or

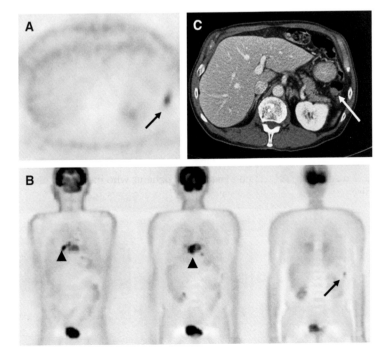

Fig. 6. (*A*, *B*) The patient had stage IIIB NSCLC (central tumor and contralateral lymph node spread) (*arrowheads*) and an FDG-avid lesion in the left upper abdomen (*arrow*). (*C*) Abdominal CT suggested a colon lesion (*arrow*) that was confirmed to be early colorectal cancer at colonoscopy.

CT) remains the method of choice to stage the brain.

Although some PET images can be considered definite proof of multifocal metastatic disease (Fig. 7), caution always is indicated in solitary extrathoracic PET findings that determine the chances for radical therapy (Fig. 8). In these patients, a confirmatory test, such as needle aspiration cytology of an adrenal gland abnormality or demonstration of osteolysis on bone imaging, is indicated.

Baseline staging: consequences of PET in the work-up of non–small cell lung cancer

Guidance of invasive procedures

In addition to CT, PET is of help in directing tissue-sampling techniques in the staging of lung cancer. This is the case for mediastinoscopy as well as for the more recent ultrasound-guided endoscopic techniques such as esophageal ultrasonography (EUS) or endobronchial ultrasonography (EBUS) with a curved linear array ultrasound transducer (Fig. 9). The advent of endoscopic ultrasonography has allowed imaging beyond the mucosa into the mediastinum.

EUS is performed with an esophageal endoscope that guides the ultrasound image through the esophageal wall toward the mediastinal LN of interest, allowing a controlled fine-needle aspiration (FNA) through the working channel of the endoscope. This technique is particularly interesting for the posterior and inferior mediastinal LNs, which fall outside the reach of mediastinoscopy. A recent review compared CT, PET, and EUS-FNA [30]. The review reported a sensitivity of 57% and a specificity of 82% for CT, of 84% and 89%, respectively, for PET, and of 78% and 71%, respectively, for EUS-FNA. Another series of consecutive patients who had suspected lung cancer on chest radiograph

compared CT, PET, and EUS-FNA [73]. PET and EUS-FNA had similar sensitivities (63% versus 68%, respectively) and similar negative predictive values (64% versus 68%, respectively), but EUS-FNA had superior specificity (100%, versus 72% for PET; $P = .004$). Another series compared the accuracy of EUS-FNA of the posterior/inferior mediastinal LN stations in patients who had had a positive PET or CT scan. The accuracy of EUS-FNA was 97%, whereas the accuracy of PET was only 50% [74]. A smaller series concentrated on EUS-FNA in patients who had positive mediastinal LNs on PET. The sensitivity, specificity, negative predictive value, positive predictive value, and accuracy of EUS-FNA in analyzing PET-positive nodes were 93%, 100%, 80%, 100%, and 94%, respectively [75].

EBUS can be performed with a bronchoscope, allowing needle aspiration of superior mediastinal, subcarinal, and hilar LNs under direct ultrasound vision (EBUS-controlled transbronchial needle aspiration [TBNA]). Only one series is available so far comparing EBUS-controlled TBNA, PET only, and thoracic CT in the detection of mediastinal and hilar LN metastasis in patients who have lung cancer considered for surgical resection. The series reported a sensitivity of 92.3%, a specificity of 100%, and diagnostic accuracy of 98% for EBUS-TBNA; of 80%, of 70.1%, and 72.5%, respectively, for PET; and of 76.9%, 55.3%, and 60.8%, respectively, for CT [76].

Impact on overall stage and management

Noninvasive lung cancer staging was improved substantially by the use of PET. The most exciting feature of PET is that it gives a reasonably cancer-specific imaging of the entire patient in one single, noninvasive test. Apart from the information on the probability of malignancy in the primary lesion, the technique is can stage both intra- and extrathoracic sites in

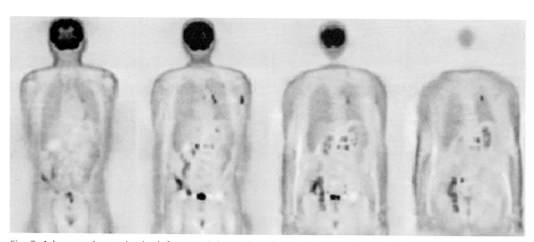

Fig. 7. Adenocarcinoma in the left upper lobe with ipsilateral adenopathy. Multiple metastatic bone lesions.

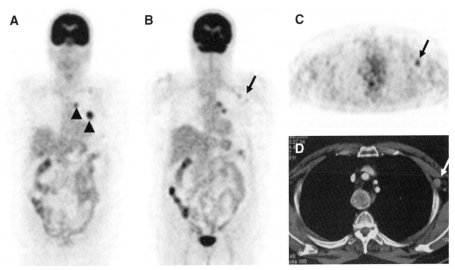

Fig. 8. (A) A 71-year-old woman who has left lung tumor with accompanying left para-aortic lymph nodes (*arrowheads*). (B, C) FDG-PET also suggested left axillary lymph node metastases (*arrow*). (D) CT showed a similar picture. Biopsy revealed inflammatory hydradenitis. With final-stage cT2N2 disease, the patient was a candidate for radical multimodality treatment.

one examination, with a better accuracy than conventional imaging and thus with a potential impact on stage designation and therapeutic decision.

For preoperative mediastinal LN staging, PET has become the most accurate noninvasive diagnostic test. The additional use of PET in preoperative or preradiation therapy staging led to a stage shift in about half (range, 19%–62%) of patients staged with conventional CT. The changes mostly involved upstaging (range, 12%–56%), less frequently involved downstaging, and were related mainly to the detection of unexpected distant lesions by PET (range, 10%–36%) [48,51–54,58,77–80]. In 19% to 46% of cases, the addition of PET imaging also resulted in a change of treatment plan, that is, a change in treatment intent (curative versus palliative), in treatment modality (surgery versus

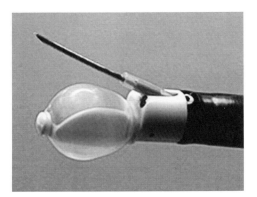

Fig. 9. Endobronchial ultrasonography bronchoscope with a curved linear array ultrasound transducer allowing real-time fine-needle aspiration.

radiotherapy), or in treatment planning (eg, field of radiotherapy) [42,46,48,51,53,54,58,77–80].

A randomized trial addressed whether PET can reduce the number of futile thoracotomies. In the Pet in Lung cancer Staging (PLUS) trial, PET added to conventional imaging strikingly reduced the number of futile thoracotomies in patients who had potentially resectable NSCLC [59]. There was a significant reduction of futile thoracotomies, from 41% in the group assessed with conventional imaging alone to 21% in the group assessed with conventional imaging plus PET, irrespective of clinical stage. Furthermore, PET did not decrease nonfutile thoracotomies (44% versus 41%), because PET improved identification of patients who would benefit from thoracotomy. On the other hand, the recent prospective POORT study illustrated that the use of PET immediately after first presentation did not reduce the overall number of diagnostic tests in comparison with traditional work-up [81]. This study had an inherent limitation in the protocol design: PET scans were not read in conjunction with CT, an approach that is known to improve the accuracy of both tests.

Small cell lung cancer

In contrast to the multitude of data on PET in NSCLC, there are far fewer studies of its accuracy in small cell lung cancer (SCLC) [82–87]. There are several possible reasons. First, SCLC now represents only 15% to 20% of all lung cancers. Second, it is a tumor with early spread into distant sites, thereby obviating the need for PET in many patients. For that reason, patients who have SCLC often are categorized as having limited disease (LD) or extensive disease (ED). According to the consensus definition of the International Association for the Study of Lung Cancer (IASLC), patients who have a tumor confined to one hemithorax including contralateral hilar and supraclavicular nodes have LD [88] These patients are candidates for radical concurrent chemoradiotherapy [89]. Patients who have ED have palliative chemotherapy only.

Regarding the main goal of baseline SCLC staging—the distinction between LD and ED—one prospective study examined how often PET detected ED SCLC in patients considered to have LD based on conventional staging [90]. PET correctly upstaged 2 of 24 patients to ED. PET also correctly depicted all tumor sites in the primary mass and nodal stations. PET impacted the radiotherapy planning by detecting unsuspected locoregional LN metastasis in 6 of 24 patients.

In the largest study to date, 91 patients who had SCLC underwent conventional staging including cranial MR imaging or CT and FDG-PET [91]. In 14 patients, PET caused a stage migration, correctly upstaging 10 patients to ED and downstaging 3 patients to LD. PET was significantly superior to CT in detecting extrathoracic metastases except for the brain.

Restaging after induction therapy

One of the greatest challenges in noninvasive staging is the optimal reassessment of tumor response after induction therapy, including the pathologic response in the primary tumor as well as the downstaging of mediastinal LNs.

The assessment of the tumor response to induction treatment usually is performed on CT imaging. A reduction in tumor volume after induction therapy is considered a predictor of pathologic tumor response. Definitive pathologic assessment of the primary tumor or mediastinal LNs, however, sometimes shows pathologic complete response or mediastinal downstaging, despite the absence of radiologic changes in the tumor volume after induction therapy. Because FDG preferentially accumulates in viable tumor cells and not in fibrotic or necrotic tissue, a change in FDG uptake on PET after induction therapy is considered a better parameter for response evaluation and restaging after induction chemotherapy.

The clinical experience with PET for the detection of residual primary tumor or mediastinal LN involvement after induction therapy for operable NSCLC is rapidly increasing. Eleven studies, most with a small number of patients, are available [92–102].

Some of these studies demonstrated that a repeat PET after induction therapy accurately detects viable tissue in the primary tumor with a sensitivity ranging from 67% to 97% [92,93,97,98]. The presence of false-positive findings in the primary tumor, especially after chemoradiotherapy, hampers the usefulness of PET scan for response evaluation after induction therapy, however.

PET is less sensitive in staging LNs after induction treatment than in the untreated patient. Six mediastinal restaging studies yield a lower sensitivity of PET, ranging from 20% to 71% [92–94,96,97]. Three prospective studies have been performed on a homogeneous group of patients who had pathology-confirmed baseline stage III NSCLC [95–97]. PET after induction chemotherapy for stage IIIA-N2 NSCLC had a sensitivity of 71% in the detection of persistent mediastinal LN disease in one group [96]; a sensitivity of 58% was reported in a study with chemoradiotherapy induction [97]. In the three other studies [92–94], only a minority of the patients had baseline pathology-proven mediastinal LN involvement. One study is difficult to interpret, because only a minority of patients underwent a baseline PET [92]. A second small, prospective study with 34 patients receiving induction chemotherapy for stage IB-IIIA NSCLC reported a disappointing sensitivity of only 50% for detection of malignant LN involvement in general but a surprisingly accurate prediction of the paratracheal N2 LN status with a sensitivity of 100% [93]. In the third small, prospective study with 25 patients, PET after induction chemotherapy for stage IB-IIIA NSCLC had a sensitivity of only 20% for pathologic mediastinal involvement [94]. Although metabolic imaging has the potential of improving the restaging of the primary tumor and mediastinum after induction therapy, its clinical role has not been well defined by the currently available data. More and larger prospective data are needed.

Very recently, two prospective trials studied the role of fusion PET-CT in stage IIIA-N2 NSCLC. A LLCG study compared the role of integrated PET-CT and re-mediastinoscopy to assess pathologic staging after induction chemotherapy. The results of re-mediastinoscopy were disappointing, but the sensitivity and specificity of integrated PET-CT were better than that of visually compared PET and CT images (77% and 92%, respectively) (Fig. 10) [96,99]. Similar results were found by Cerfolio and colleagues [100], although the nature of the study was different. Fusion PET-CT and repeated CT were compared with definitive pathologic staging after induction chemoradiotherapy. A statistical significance in direct comparison was achieved in favor of integrated PET-CT.

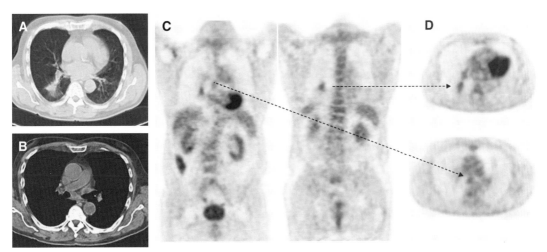

Fig. 10. A patient who has stage IIIA-N2 disease. After induction chemotherapy, (*A*) the primary tumor in the right lung and (*B*) the subcarinal adenopathy have decreased in size. On (*C*) coronal and (*D*) transaxial PET images, moderate FDG uptake is still present in the primary and in the subcarinal space. Endoscopic needle aspiration confirmed persistent N2 disease.

Pitfalls in staging lung cancer with PET

False-negative findings

A critical mass of metabolically active malignant cells is required for PET detection of a neoplastic site. LN and distant staging results with PET should be interpreted with caution in tumors with decreased FDG uptake, such as very well-differentiated adenocarcinoma, bronchoalveolar carcinoma, or carcinoid tumors. Furthermore, factors inherent to the technique, such as perivenous FDG injection, or high baseline glucose serum levels should be taken into account.

False-positive findings

FDG uptake is not specific for malignancy, and false-positive findings can occur in any part of the body that has increased glucose metabolic activity (Box 1). Infections and inflammatory conditions, such as bacterial pneumonia [103] or pyogenic abscess, or aspergillosis and granulomatous diseases, such as active sarcoidosis [104], tuberculosis, histoplasmosis, coccidiomycosis, Wegener's disease, and coal miner's lung, are the most common conditions. In these lesions, the FDG uptake has been attributed to an increase in granulocyte or macrophage activity [105]. Recently, brown fat gained attention as a possible cause of benign FDG uptake. Brown fat usually has a bilateral and symmetric distribution but may be asymmetric and focal. Because this uptake may occur in regions of potential malignant LN spread (cervical, supraclavicular, axillary, mediastinal, and abdominal regions), the differential diagnosis may be difficult

Box 1: Possible false-positive findings on PET for lung cancer

Infections
(Postobstructive) pneumonia
Mycobacterial or fungal infection

Inflammatory conditions
Granulomatous disorders (eg, sarcoidosis, Wegener disease)
Chronic nonspecific lymphadenitis
(Rheumatoid) arthritis
Occupational (anthracosilicosis)
Reflux esophagitis
Nonspecific (bronchiectasis, organizing pneumonia)

Iatrogenic causes
Radiation esophagitis
Radiation pneumonitis
Bone marrow hyperplasia after chemotherapy
Colony-stimulating factors
Invasive procedures (lymph node or lung biopsy; thoracocentesis; chest tube)

Physiologic causes
Muscle activity
Unilateral vocal cord activity (paralysis other side)
Aortic wall (atherosclerotic plaque)
Brown fat

Benign mass lesions
Salivary gland adenoma–Whartin tumor
Thyroid adenoma
Adrenal adenoma
Colorectal dysplastic polyp

when PET images are interpreted without the aid of CT images. In most instances, correlation with CT images, preferably by PET-CT fusion images, can resolve the problem [106].

References

[1] Schrevens L, Lorent N, Dooms C, et al. The role of PET-scan in diagnosis, staging and management of non-small cell lung cancer. Oncologist 2004;9:633–43.

[2] Vansteenkiste J, Fischer BM, Dooms C, et al. Positron-emission tomography in prognostic and therapeutic assessment of lung cancer: systematic review. Lancet Oncol 2004;5:531–40.

[3] Mountain CF. Revisions in the international system for staging lung cancer. Chest 1997;111(6): 1710–7.

[4] Naruke T, Suemasu K, Ishikawa S. Lymph node mapping and curability at various levels of metastasis in resected lung cancer. J Thorac Cardiovasc Surg 1978;76:832–7.

[5] American Thoracic Society (ATS). Clinical staging of primary lung cancer. Am Rev Respir Dis 1983;127:1–11.

[6] Mountain CF, Dresler CM. Regional lymph node classification for lung cancer staging. Chest 1997;111(6):1718–23.

[7] Vansteenkiste J, Dooms C, Becker H, et al. Multimodality treatment of stage III non-small cell lung cancer: staging procedures. Eur J Cancer 2005;3(Suppl 3):7–19.

[8] Arriagada R, Bergman B, Dunant A, et al, for the International Adjuvant Lung Cancer Trial Collaborative Group. Cisplatin-based adjuvant chemotherapy in patients with completely resected non-small cell lung cancer. N Engl J Med 2004; 350:351–60.

[9] Jett JR, Scott WJ, Rivera MP, et al. Guidelines on treatment of stage IIIB non-small cell lung cancer. Chest 2003;123(Suppl 1):221S–5S.

[10] Vansteenkiste J, De Leyn P, Deneffe G, et al. Present status of induction treatment for N2 non-small cell lung cancer: a review. Eur J Cardiothorac Surg 1998;13:1–12.

[11] Rosell R, Gomez Codina J, Camps C, et al. A randomized trial comparing preoperative chemotherapy plus surgery with surgery alone in patients with non-small-cell lung cancer. N Engl J Med 1994;330:153–8.

[12] Betticher DC, Hsu Schmitz SF, Totsch M, et al. Mediastinal lymph node clearance after docetaxel-cisplatin neoadjuvant chemotherapy is prognostic of survival in patients with stage IIIA pN2 non-small cell lung cancer: a multicenter phase II trial. J Clin Oncol 2003;21:1752–9.

[13] Lorent N, De Leyn P, Lievens Y, et al. Long-term survival of surgically staged IIIA-N2 non-small cell lung cancer treated with surgical combined modality approach: analysis of a 7-year experience. Ann Oncol 2004;15:1645–53.

[14] Vansteenkiste JF, Vandebroek JE, Nackaerts KL, et al. Clinical benefit response in advanced non-small cell lung cancer. A multicenter prospective randomized phase III study of single agent gemcitabine versus cisplatin-vindesine. Ann Oncol 2001;12:1221–30.

[15] Numico G, Russi E, Merlano M. Best supportive care in non-small cell lung cancer: is there a role for radiotherapy and chemotherapy? Lung Cancer 2001;32:213–26.

[16] Bittner RC, Felix R. Magnetic resonance (MR) imaging of the chest: state-of-the-art. Eur Respir J 1998;11:1392–404.

[17] Glazer HS, Kaiser LR, Anderson DJ, et al. Indeterminate mediastinal invasion in bronchogenic carcinoma: CT evaluation. Radiology 1989; 173(1):37–42.

[18] Kameda K, Adachi S, Kono M. Detection of T-factor in lung cancer using magnetic resonance imaging and computed tomography. J Thorac Imaging 1988;3(2):73–80.

[19] Izbicki JR, Thetter O, Karg O, et al. Accuracy of computed tomographic scan and surgical assessment for staging of bronchial carcinoma. A prospective study. J Thorac Cardiovasc Surg 1992;104(2):413–20.

[20] Hierholzer J, Luo L, Bittner RC, et al. MRI and CT in the differential diagnosis of pleural disease. Chest 2000;118(3):604–9.

[21] Pearlberg JL, Sandler MA, Beute GH, et al. Limitations of CT in evaluation of neoplasms involving chest wall. J Comput Assist Tomogr 1987;11(2):290–3.

[22] Lardinois D, Weder W, Hany TF, et al. Staging of non-small cell lung cancer with integrated positron-emission tomography and computed tomography. N Engl J Med 2003;348:2500–7.

[23] De Wever W, Ceyssens S, Mortelmans L, et al. Additional value of PET-CT in the staging of lung cancer: comparison with CT alone, PET alone and visual correlation of PET and CT. Eur Radiol 2006.

[24] Erasmus JJ, McAdams HP, Rossi SE, et al. FDG PET of pleural effusions in patients with non-small cell lung cancer. AJR Am J Roentgenol 2000;175:245–9.

[25] Gupta NC, Rogers JS, Graeber GM, et al. Clinical role of F-18 fluorodeoxyglucose positron emission tomography imaging in patients with lung cancer and suspected malignant pleural effusion. Chest 2002;122:1918–24.

[26] Schaffler GJ, Wolf G, Schoellnast H, et al. Non-small cell lung cancer: evaluation of pleural abnormalities on CT scans with 18F FDG PET. Radiology 2004;231:858–65.

[27] Shim SS, Lee KS, Kim BT, et al. Integrated PET/CT and the dry pleural dissemination of peripheral adenocarcinoma of the lung: diagnostic implications. J Comput Assist Tomogr 2006; 30:70–6.

[28] Martini N, Kris MG, Ginsberg RJ. The role of multimodality therapy in locoregional

non-small cell lung cancer. Surg Oncol Clin N Am 1997;6:769–91.

[29] Dillemans B, Deneffe G, Verschakelen J, et al. Value of computed tomography and mediastinoscopy in preoperative evaluation of mediastinal nodes in non-small cell lung cancer. Eur J Cardiothorac Surg 1994;8:37–42.

[30] Toloza EM, Harpole L, McCrory DC. Noninvasive staging of non-small cell lung cancer: a review of the current evidence. Chest 2003; 123(Suppl 1):137S–46S.

[31] Vansteenkiste JF, Stroobants SG, De Leyn PR, et al. Lymph node staging in non-small cell lung cancer with FDG-PET scan: a prospective study on 690 lymph node stations from 68 patients. J Clin Oncol 1998;16:2142–9.

[32] Dwamena BA, Sonnad SS, Angobaldo JO, et al. Metastases from non-small cell lung cancer: mediastinal staging in the 1990s. Meta-analytic comparison of PET and CT. Radiology 1999; 213:530–6.

[33] Fischer BM, Mortensen J, Hojgaard L. Positron emission tomography in the diagnosis and staging of lung cancer: a systematic, quantitative review. Lancet Oncol 2001;2:659–66.

[34] Hellwig D, Ukena D, Paulsen F, et al. Meta-analysis of the efficacy of positron emission tomography with F-18-fluorodeoxyglucose in lung tumors. Basis for discussion of the German Consensus Conference on PET in Oncology 2000 (in German). Pneumologie 2001;55:367–77.

[35] Gould MK, Kuschner WG, Rydzak CE, et al. Test performance of positron emission tomography and computed tomography for mediastinal staging in patients with non-small cell lung cancer: a meta-analysis. Ann Intern Med 2003; 139:879–92.

[36] Gupta NC, Graeber GM, Bishop HA. Comparative efficacy of positron emission tomography with fluorodeoxyglucose in evaluation of small (3 cm) lymph node lesions. Chest 2000;117(3): 773–8.

[37] Vansteenkiste JF. FDG-PET for lymph node staging in NSCLC: a major step forward, but beware of the pitfalls. [editorial]. Lung Cancer 2005;47: 151–3.

[38] Takamochi K, Yoshida J, Murakami K, et al. Pitfalls in lymph node staging with positron emission tomography in non-small cell lung cancer patients. Lung Cancer 2005;47:235–42.

[39] Vansteenkiste JF, De Leyn PR, Deneffe GJ, et al. Survival and prognostic factors in resected N2 non-small cell lung cancer: a study of 140 cases. The Leuven Lung Cancer Group. Ann Thorac Surg 1997;63:1441–50.

[40] Bollen EC, Theunissen PH, Van Duin CJ, et al. Clinical significance of intranodal and extranodal growth in lymph node metastases of non-small cell lung cancer. Scand J Thorac Cardiovasc Surg 1994;28:97–102.

[41] Vansteenkiste JF, Stroobants SG, De Leyn PR, et al. Mediastinal lymph node staging with FDG-PET scan in patients with potentially operable non-small cell lung cancer: a prospective analysis of 50 cases. Chest 1997;112:1480–6.

[42] Weng E, Tran L, Rege S, et al. Accuracy and clinical impact of mediastinal lymph node staging with FDG-PET imaging in potentially resectable lung cancer. Am J Clin Oncol 2000;23(1): 47–52.

[43] Fritscher-Ravens A, Bohuslavizki KH, Brandt L, et al. Mediastinal lymph node involvement in potentially resectable lung cancer: comparison of CT, positron emission tomography, and endoscopic ultrasonography with and without fine-needle aspiration. Chest 2003;123:442–51.

[44] Quint LE, Tummala S, Brisson LJ, et al. Distribution of distant metastases from newly diagnosed non- small cell lung cancer. Ann Thorac Surg 1996;62(1):246–50.

[45] Pantel K, Izbicki J, Passlick B, et al. Frequency and prognostic significance of isolated tumour cells in bone marrow of patients with non-small cell lung cancer without overt metastases. Lancet 1996;347(9002):649–53.

[46] Lewis P, Griffin S, Marsden P, et al. Whole-body 18F-fluorodeoxyglucose positron emission tomography in preoperative evaluation of lung cancer. Lancet 1994;344:1265–6.

[47] Valk PE, Pounds TR, Hopkins DM, et al. Staging non-small cell lung cancer by whole-body positron emission tomographic imaging. Ann Thorac Surg 1995;60(6):1573–81.

[48] Bury T, Dowlati A, Paulus P, et al. Whole-body 18FDG positron emission tomography in the staging of non-small cell lung cancer. Eur Respir J 1997;10:2529–34.

[49] Weder W, Schmid RA, Bruchhaus H, et al. Detection of extrathoracic metastases by positron emission tomography in lung cancer. Ann Thorac Surg 1998;66(3):886–92.

[50] Marom EM, McAdams HP, Erasmus JJ, et al. Staging non-small cell lung cancer with whole-body PET. Radiology 1999;212(3):803–9.

[51] Saunders CA, Dussek JE, O'Doherty MJ, et al. Evaluation of fluorine-18-fluorodeoxyglucose whole body positron emission tomography imaging in the staging of lung cancer. Ann Thorac Surg 1999;67(3):790–7.

[52] Pieterman RM, Van Putten JW, Meuzelaar JJ, et al. Preoperative staging of non-small cell lung cancer with positron emission tomography. N Engl J Med 2000;343:254–61.

[53] Mac Manus MP, Hicks RJ, Matthews JP, et al. High rate of detection of unsuspected distant metastases by PET in apparent stage III non-small cell lung cancer: implications for radical radiation therapy. Int J Radiat Oncol Biol Phys 2001;50:287–93.

[54] Hicks RJ, Kalff V, Mac Manus MP, et al. 18F-FDG PET provides high-impact and powerful prognostic stratification in staging newly diagnosed non-small cell lung cancer. J Nucl Med 2001;42:1596–604.

[55] Eschmann SM, Friedel G, Paulsen F, et al. FDG PET for staging of advanced non-small cell lung cancer prior to neoadjuvant radio-chemotherapy. Eur J Nucl Med Mol Imaging 2002;29: 804–8.

[56] Vesselle H, Pugsley JM, Vallieres E, et al. The impact of fluorodeoxyglucose F18 positron emission tomography on the surgical staging of non-small cell lung cancer. J Thorac Cardiovasc Surg 2002;124:511–9.

[57] Stroobants S, Dhoore I, Dooms C, et al. Additional value of whole-body fluorodeoxyglucose positron emission tomography in the detection of distant metastases of non-small cell lung cancer. Clin Lung Cancer 2003;4:242–7.

[58] Hoekstra CJ, Stroobants SG, Hoekstra OS, et al. The value of [18F]fluoro-2-deoxy-D-glucose positron emission tomography in the selection of patients with stage IIIA-N2 non-small cell lung cancer for combined modality treatment. Lung Cancer 2003;39:151–7.

[59] Van Tinteren H, Hoekstra OS, Smit EF, et al. Effectiveness of positron emission tomography in the preoperative assessment of patients with suspected non-small cell lung cancer: the PLUS multicentre randomised trial. Lancet 2002; 359:1388–93.

[60] Erasmus JJ, Patz EF, McAdams HP, et al. Evaluation of adrenal masses in patients with bronchogenic carcinoma using 18F-fluorodeoxyglucose positron emission tomography. AJR Am J Roentgenol 1997;168(5):1357–60.

[61] Boland GW, Goldberg MA, Lee MJ, et al. Indeterminate adrenal mass in patients with cancer: evaluation at PET with 2-[F-18]-fluoro-2-deoxy-D-glucose. Radiology 1995;194(1):131–4.

[62] Yun M, Kim W, Alnafisi N, et al. 18F-FDG PET in characterizing adrenal lesions detected on CT or MRI. J Nucl Med 2001;42:1795–7.

[63] Oliver TW, Bernardino ME, Miller JI, et al. Isolated adrenal masses in non-small cell bronchogenic carcinoma. Radiology 1984;153(1): 217–8.

[64] Ettinghausen SE, Burt ME. Prospective evaluation of unilateral adrenal masses in patients with operable non-small cell lung cancer. J Clin Oncol 1991;9(8):1462–6.

[65] Bury T, Barreto A, Daenen F, et al. Fluorine-18 deoxyglucose positron emission tomography for the detection of bone metastases in patients with non-small cell lung cancer. Eur J Nucl Med 1998;25(9):1244–7.

[66] Hsia TC, Shen YY, Yen RF, et al. Comparing whole body 18F-2-deoxyglucose positron emission tomography and technetium-99m methylene diophosphate bone scan to detect bone metastases in patients with non-small cell lung cancer. Neoplasma 2002;49:267–71.

[67] Gayed I, Vu T, Johnson M, et al. Comparison of bone and 2-deoxy-2-[18F]fluoro-D-glucose positron emission tomography in the evaluation of bony metastases in lung cancer. Mol Imaging Biol 2003;5:26–31.

[68] Cheran SK, Herndon JE, Patz EF. Comparison of whole-body FDG-PET to bone scan for detection of bone metastases in patients with a new diagnosis of lung cancer. Lung Cancer 2004;44: 317–25.

[69] Kao CH, Hsieh JF, Tsai SC, et al. Comparison and discrepancy of 18F-2-deoxyglucose positron emission tomography and Tc-99m MDP bone scan to detect bone metastases. Anticancer Res 2000;20(3B):2189–92.

[70] Cook GJ, Houston S, Rubens R, et al. Detection of bone metastases in breast cancer by 18FDG PET: differing metabolic activity in osteoblastic and osteolytic lesions. J Clin Oncol 1998; 16(10):3375–9.

[71] Hustinx R, Paulus P, Jacquet N, et al. Clinical evaluation of whole-body 18F-fluorodeoxyglucose positron emission tomography in the detection of liver metastases. Ann Oncol 1998; 9(4):397–401.

[72] Delbeke D, Martin WH, Sandler MP, et al. Evaluation of benign vs malignant hepatic lesions with positron emission tomography. Arch Surg 1998;133(5):510–5.

[73] Fritscher-Ravens A, Davidson BL, Hauber HP, et al. Endoscopic ultrasound, positron emission tomography, and computerized tomography for lung cancer. Am J Respir Crit Care Med 2003;168: 1293–7.

[74] Eloubeidi MA, Cerfolio RJ, Chen VK, et al. Endoscopic ultrasound-guided fine needle aspiration of mediastinal lymph node in patients with suspected lung cancer after positron emission tomography and computed tomography scans. Ann Thorac Surg 2005;79:263–8.

[75] Annema JT, Hoekstra OS, Smit EF, et al. Towards a minimally invasive staging strategy in NSCLC: analysis of PET positive mediastinal lesions by EUS-FNA. Lung Cancer 2004;44:53–60.

[76] Yasufuku K, Nakajima T, Motoori K, et al. Comparison of endobronchial ultrasound, positron emission tomography, and CT for lymph node staging of lung cancer. Chest 2006;130(3):710–8.

[77] Vanuytsel LJ, Vansteenkiste JF, Stroobants SG, et al. The impact of (18)F-fluoro-2-deoxy-D-glucose positron emission tomography (FDG-PET) lymph node staging on the radiation treatment volumes in patients with non-small cell lung cancer. Radiother Oncol 2000;55: 317–24.

[78] Kalff V, Hicks RJ, Mac Manus M, et al. Clinical impact of (18)F-fluorodeoxyglucose positron emission tomography in patients with non-small cell lung cancer: A prospective study. J Clin Oncol 2001;19:111–8.

[79] Changlai SP, Tsai SC, Chou MC, et al. Whole body 18F-2-deoxyglucose positron emission tomography to restage non-small cell lung cancer. Oncol Rep 2001;8:337–9.

[80] Dizendorf EV, Baumert BG, Von Schulthess GK, et al. Impact of whole-body 18F-FDG PET on staging and managing patients for radiation therapy. J Nucl Med 2003;44:24–9.

[81] Herder GJ, Kramer H, Hoekstra OS, et al. Traditional versus up-front [18F] fluorodeoxyglucose positron emission tomography staging of non-small cell lung cancer: a Dutch cooperative randomized study. J Clin Oncol 2006;24(12): 1800–6.

[82] Schumacher T, Brink I, Mix M, et al. FDG-PET imaging for the staging and follow-up of small cell lung cancer. Eur J Nucl Med 2001;28:483–8.

[83] Chin R, McCain TW, Miller AA, et al. Whole body FDG-PET for the evaluation and staging of small cell lung cancer: a preliminary study. Lung Cancer 2002;37:1–6.

[84] Shen YY, Shiau YC, Wang JJ, et al. Whole-body 18F-2-deoxyglucose positron emission tomography in primary staging small cell lung cancer. Anticancer Res 2002;22:1257–64.

[85] Zhao DS, Valdivia AY, Li Y, et al. 18F-fluoro-deoxyglucose positron emission tomography in small cell lung cancer. Semin Nucl Med 2002;32:272–5.

[86] Kamel EM, Zwahlen D, Wyss MT, et al. Whole-body 18F-FDG PET improves the management of patients with small cell lung cancer. J Nucl Med 2003;44:1911–7.

[87] Blum R, Mac Manus MP, Rischin D, et al. Impact of positron emission tomography on the management of patients with small cell lung cancer: preliminary experience. Am J Clin Oncol 2004;27:164–71.

[88] Micke P, Faldum A, Metz T, et al. Staging small cell lung cancer: Veterans Administration Lung Study Group versus International Association for the Study of Lung Cancer—what limits limited disease? Lung Cancer 2002;37:271–6.

[89] De Ruysscher D, Vansteenkiste J. Chest radiotherapy in limited stage small cell lung cancer: facts, questions, prospects. Radiother Oncol 2000;55:1–9.

[90] Bradley JD, Dehdashti F, Mintun MA, et al. Positron emission tomography in limited-stage small cell lung cancer: a prospective study. J Clin Oncol 2004;22:3248–54.

[91] Brink I, Schumacher T, Mix M, et al. Impact of 18F-FDG-PET on the primary staging of small cell lung cancer. Eur J Nucl Med Mol Imaging 2005;31:1614–20.

[92] Akhurst T, Downey RJ, Ginsberg MS, et al. An initial experience with FDG-PET in the imaging of residual disease after induction therapy for lung cancer. Ann Thorac Surg 2002;73:259–66.

[93] Cerfolio RJ, Ojha B, Mukherjee S, et al. Positron emission tomography scanning with 2-fluoro-2-deoxy-d- glucose as a predictor of response of neoadjuvant treatment for non-small cell carcinoma. J Thorac Cardiovasc Surg 2003;125: 938–44.

[94] Port JL, Kent MS, Korst RJ, et al. Positron emission tomography scanning poorly predicts response to preoperative chemotherapy in non-small cell lung cancer. Ann Thorac Surg 2004;77:254–9.

[95] Vansteenkiste JF, Stroobants SG, De Leyn PR, et al. Potential use of FDG-PET scan after induction chemotherapy in surgically staged IIIA-N2 non-small cell lung cancer: a prospective pilot study. Ann Oncol 1998;9:1193–8.

[96] Vansteenkiste J, Stroobants S, Hoekstra C, et al. 18fluoro-2-deoxyglucose positron emission tomography (PET) in the assessment of induction chemotherapy (IC) in stage IIIA-N2 NSCLC: a multi-center prospective study. Proc Am Soc Clin Oncol 2001;20:313A.

[97] Ryu JS, Choi NC, Fischman AJ, et al. FDG-PET in staging and restaging non-small cell lung cancer after neoadjuvant chemoradiotherapy: correlation with histopathology. Lung Cancer 2002;35:179–87.

[98] Choi NC, Fischman AJ, Niemierko A, et al. Dose-response relationship between probability of pathologic tumor control and glucose metabolic rate measured with FDG PET after preoperative chemoradiotherapy in locally advanced non-small cell lung cancer. Int J Radiat Oncol Biol Phys 2002;54:1024–35.

[99] De Leyn P, Stroobants S, De Wever W, et al. Prospective comparative study of integrated positron emission tomography-computed tomography compared with remediastinoscopy in the assessment of residual mediastinal lymph node disease after induction chemotherapy for mediastinoscopy proven stage IIIA-N2 non-small cell lung cancer: A Leuven Lung Cancer Group study. J Clin Oncol 2006;24:3333–9.

[100] Cerfolio RJ, Bryant AS, Ojha B. Restaging patients with N2 (stage IIIa) non-small cell lung cancer after neoadjuvant chemoradiotherapy: a prospective study. J Thorac Cardiovasc Surg 2006;131(6):1229–35.

[101] Hoekstra CJ, Stroobants SG, Smit EF, et al. Prognostic relevance of response evaluation using [18F]-2-fluoro-2-deoxy-D-glucose positron emission tomography in patients with locally advanced non-small cell lung cancer. J Clin Oncol 2005;23:8362–70.

[102] Ohtsuka T, Nomori H, Ebihara A, et al. FDG-PET imaging for lymph node staging and pathologic tumor response after neoadjuvant treatment of non-small cell lung cancer. Ann Thorac Cardiovasc Surg 2006;12(2):89–94.

[103] Kapucu LO, Meltzer CC, Townsend DW, et al. Fluorine-18-fluorodeoxyglucose uptake in pneumonia. J Nucl Med 1998;39(7):1267–9.

[104] Brudin LH, Valind SO, Rhodes CG, et al. Fluorine-18 deoxyglucose uptake in sarcoidosis measured with positron emission tomography. Eur J Nucl Med 1994;21(4):297–305.

[105] Bakheet SM, Saleem M, Powe J, et al. F-18 fluorodeoxyglucose chest uptake in lung inflammation and infection. Clin Nucl Med 2000;25(4): 273–8.

[106] Truong MT, Erasmus JJ, Munden RF, et al. Focal FDG uptake in mediastinal brown fat mimicking malignancy: a potential pitfall resolved on PET/CT. AJR Am J Roentgenol 2004;183:1127–32.

ELSEVIER
SAUNDERS

POSITRON
EMISSION
TOMOGRAPHY

PET Clin 1 (2006) 317–328

Impact of PET on Radiation Therapy Planning

Michael P. Mac Manus, MD, MRCP, FRCR, FFRRCSI, FRANZCR[a],*,
Rodney J. Hicks, MD, FRACP[b]

Of all the medical disciplines, radiation oncology could well be the clinical specialty most dependent on accurate three-dimensional imaging. Unlike an oncological surgeon who may modify his or her assessment of the extent of disease during an operation, the radiation oncologist is usually reliant on imaging to guide the entire treatment process, albeit supplemented by pathology reports, clinical examination, and other information depending upon the clinical situation. To direct a tumoricidal dose of radiation to a tumor, while sparing normal tissues as much as possible, the precise spatial location of the primary tumor and of tumor-bearing lymph nodes must be appreciated, together with the anatomy of the critical adjacent normal tissues.

A perfect radiation therapy (RT) plan would deliver a lethal dose to the tumor and no dose at all to the normal tissues. Such perfection is of course unattainable with the photon beams produced by linear accelerators, although proton beams may provide a closer approximation [1]. Nevertheless, the use of multiple, carefully shaped and modulated photon beams can produce remarkably good results, but only if treatment is directed to precisely the right location in three-dimensional space.

In the last decade or so, rapid improvements in the technology available for RT planning and delivery have occurred and future developments are likely [2]. Extraordinarily advanced treatment planning systems now allow much more accurate and

a Department of Radiation Oncology, Peter MacCallum Cancer Centre, St Andrew's Place, East Melbourne, Vic 3002, Australia
b Centre for Molecular Imaging, Peter MacCallum Cancer Centre, 12 Cathedral Place, East Melbourne, Vic 3002, Australia
* Corresponding author.
E-mail address: mmanus@petermac.unimelb.edu.au (M.P. Mac Manus).

doi:10.1016/j.cpet.2006.09.002

rapid three-dimensional radiation dose calculations with quantitative volumetric assessment of dose both to tumor and critical normal tissues [3]. This new complexity in dose calculation has been accompanied by an increased ability to accurately deliver ionizing radiation to complex three-dimensional shapes, using linear accelerators with independently controlled multileaf collimators that can dynamically shape the beam of radiation during the course of treatment delivery [4]. New types of highly conformal radiotherapy such as intensity-modulated radiotherapy have become available [5], making it possible to safely escalate the radiation dose without increased toxicity as in prostate cancer [6], or to maintain existing local control rates with reduced toxicity as in head and neck cancer [7], where new parotid-sparing techniques can often avoid permanent xerostomia.

The relationships between increasing radiation dose and tumor control and increasing radiation dose and the probability of a serious complication of treatment are classically described by paired sigmoid curves (Fig. 1). The greater the separation between the tumor control and radiation toxicity curves, the more likely the patient is to achieve uncomplicated local "cure" of their tumor. As a result of relative sparing of normal tissues, the newer more highly conformal RT techniques are capable of increasing the "therapeutic ratio." For a given dose of radiation prescribed to control a tumor, the ratio between the probability of tumor control and the probability of a significant complication is increased. Improving the therapeutic ratio is a key goal of research in radiation oncology.

The more highly conformal RT planning methods, with requirements for tight margins around disease sites, depend especially critically on an accurate assessment of the location of tumor sites in relation to the anatomy of normal tissues. The basis for RT planning has long been the CT scan. CT not only provides important three-dimensional anatomic information, but also provides the basis for radiation dosimetry by reconstruction of a three-dimensional electron-density map that is crucial for calculating radiation absorption and scatter. CT will remain the basis for dose calculation in radiation oncology but the information that it can provide about the location of the tumor is often insufficient by itself to accurately guide treatment. To successfully image a neoplastic lesion on CT, there must be sufficient contrast between the lesion and normal tissues. When tumors have similar imaging characteristics to surrounding normal tissues, which is often the case for lesions in the liver or spleen, they may be completely invisible on CT. Consequently, when CT is used to guide curative RT in such cases, geographic miss and ultimate treatment failure may be inevitable. Failure to image the boundary between tumor and atelectatic lung is also a common problem for the radiation oncologist relying on CT for treating lung cancer and may lead to unnecessary irradiation of large volumes of collapsed lung to avoid a geographic miss. Accurate lymph node staging is crucial for treating locoregionally advanced cancers with curative intent [8,9]. CT scanning often performs relatively poorly in this respect too because nodal size is the usual criterion for deciding if tumor is present or absent. Small nodes, negative by CT criteria, often contain tumor and benign reactive lymphadenopathy can commonly give rise to false positives in a variety of cancer sites. A good example of this

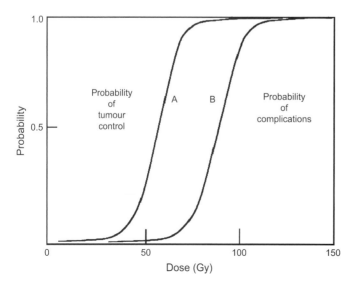

Fig. 1. Typical paired sigmoid dose-response curves for tumor control (*A*) and normal tissue complications (*B*).

phenomenon is the notoriously poor sensitivity and specificity reported in numerous clinico-pathological studies of staging the mediastinum in potentially resectable non–small cell lung cancer (NSCLC) [10].

It is fortuitous that, just when dramatic advances in RT technology were being made, a revolution was also occurring in cancer imaging with the advent of clinical PET. Staging with PET, primarily using ^{18}F-fluorodeoxyglucose (FDG) as the tracer, has rapidly acquired a key role in the management of cancers such as NSCLC [11,12], Hodgkin and non-Hodgkin lymphomas [13,14], head and neck cancers, esophageal cancers [15,16], and cervical carcinomas [17,18]. FDG-PET shows great promise in malignant melanoma [19,20], soft tissue sarcoma [21], gastrointestinal cancers [22], and a range of less common neoplasms [23,24]. Other PET tracers have the potential to image lower grade tumors when FDG is less helpful (eg, ^{18}F-labeled fluoroethylcholine in low grade glioma [25]), to identify lesions that are actively proliferating (as with ^{18}F-labeled fluorothymidine [26]), or to identify tumors with radioresistant hypoxic tumors using ^{18}F-labeled misondazole [27].

The new information provided by FDG-PET staging has the potential to immediately improve the results of radical RT by way of better selection of patients. Significantly improved survival has already been demonstrated in patients who have NSCLC selected for radical RT using PET compared with a conventionally staged control group [28], largely because patients who have PET-detected metastases and advanced locoregional disease were denied futile aggressive therapy. Incorporation of PET information into the RT planning process also has the potential to improve targeting of RT by accurately imaging regions of tumor in three dimensions [29]. A revolution in radiotherapy planning is occurring, as ways of incorporating new functional imaging data are continually being sought. In the following sections the role of PET in RT planning will be discussed in more detail.

Importance of imaging in the radiotherapy planning process

The three-dimensional radiotherapy planning process

As discussed above, the primary tool for planning curative RT is cross-sectional imaging with a CT scan. When it has been decided that a patient should receive radical RT, a treatment planning CT scan is performed with the patient in the radiotherapy treatment position with appropriate immobilization devices fitted so that patient positioning is identical for CT imaging, simulation (if performed separately), and for treatment. CT data are imported into the treatment planning software and areas of tumor are identified and contoured by the radiation oncologist using a pointing device on individual CT slices. This process generates a gross tumor volume (GTV) [30]. Normal tissues are also contoured on individual slices so that volumes of important dose-limiting organs exposed to radiation can be assessed quantitatively.

The volume that actually needs to be treated in radical RT is of course greater than the GTV because additional margins must be applied. These margins allow for a range of factors including microscopic extension of disease beyond the imaged tumor, variability in the accuracy of patient set-up on each day of treatment, and movement of the tumor (eg, with respiration). The margins applied to the GTV are disease and site specific. The volume that the radiation oncologist decides to treat, and that incorporates all of the margins around the GTV, is known as the planning target volume (PTV). The PTV is often an expansion of the GTV, generated automatically by the treatment planning software. An ideal PTV should include all gross and microscopic tumor (or at least microscopic tumor that will not be eliminated by systemic therapy) and be large enough to accommodate movement of the tumor during treatment ("internal target volume" [31]).

The next step in the process is to try to find the optimum arrangement of beams to effectively administer the prescribed radiation dose to the GTV. A variable number of individually shaped and modulated beams is applied from a range of carefully chosen angles. The range of possible solutions to a given planning problem is infinite. An ideal treatment plan would treat all parts of the PTV to the prescribed dose without exposing any healthy normal tissues to radiation. The best available RT treatment plan is one that most closely approximates this ideal and can actually be delivered in a clinical setting. Efforts are made to ensure that the inevitable dose delivered to normal tissues is "dumped" in regions where it will do least harm.

The most important step in the process, and upon which all subsequent steps depend, is the determination of the GTV. If the location of gross tumor in three-dimensional space is not accurately known and a geographic miss occurs, then treatment will be a toxic and futile exercise. Incorporation of PET into the treatment planning process has the potential to make determination of the GTV much more accurate and therefore reduce the risk of futile therapy. It is acknowledged that PET information is far from perfect. Yet for many tumor types, PET provides such a significant increase in accuracy of assessment of tumor extent that failure to use it, if available, would mean denying the patient the best possible treatment plan.

Incorporation of PET information into radiation therapy planning

In the years since the introduction of clinical PET, its importance as a tool for RT planning has become increasingly recognized. Manufacturers have become aware of the need to accommodate the ability to import and display PET information in radiotherapy planning systems. They have produced systems of increasing utility and sophistication, with the most up-to-date systems capable of allowing seamless integration of PET-CT information into the RT contouring workstation. When PET and CT imaging are combined for radiotherapy planning, the aim is to produce a biological target volume [32], incorporating all available structural and functional imaging. For lung cancer and several other malignancies, treatment of the biological target volume represents the best target for high-dose irradiation that we can currently define.

Visual incorporation of PET data into treatment planning

When clinical PET first became available to oncologists, there were no readily available means for incorporating PET information directly into the treatment planning process. Typically, PET and diagnostic CT images were simply displayed side by side on a light box and the radiation oncologist would visually incorporate the PET information when contouring the GTV. For example, if an axillary lymph node was well visualized on the planning CT and was considered uninvolved by size criteria (usually short axis diameter less than 1 cm), it would not normally be contoured as part of the GTV. If the same node, however, was identified as being FDG-avid on a PET scan and was considered to contain tumor, the node would be contoured as part of the GTV despite being negative on size criteria. In our own early prospective lung cancer study, we used this method to incorporate PET into the planning process, without any form of image coregistration. This method works quite well for small anatomically discrete structures that are easily seen on CT, but it is not a good method for helping to delineate the boundaries of larger tumors where the margins are not well imaged on CT, such as the interface between a lung tumor and atelectasis. For that purpose it was necessary to devise some method for displaying PET and CT information simultaneously within the treatment planning software.

Coregistration of separately acquired PET and CT images for treatment planning

To make full use of the three-dimensional imaging information contained in the PET scan, a number of methods were tried at different institutions before manufacturers provided commercial software and hardware solutions to make the process easy. At our own center and at other centers, in-house methods were developed for the purpose of importing PET information into the radiotherapy treatment planning system. We developed a system that used fiducial markers that were applied to the patient at separate CT and PET image acquisitions [33]. For both scans, patients were positioned identically by radiation therapists using lasers installed in both the CT and PET suites. Phantom studies showed that the method was highly reproducible and could be used in clinical practice. Digital imaging and communications in medicine PET information was imported into the radiotherapy planning system (Cadplan, Varian Medical Systems Inc., Palo Alto, California) and displayed side by side with the corresponding CT image, using software developed at our own institution. This proved highly successful in practice but, with the installation of our first combined PET/CT scanner, it has since been entirely superseded.

PET/CT for treatment planning

The optimum dataset for radiotherapy planning is provided by a modern combined PET/CT scanner. PET and CT images are acquired on the same gantry, without the need for repositioning the patient. This represents a major advance on older methods. PET/CT is not available at all centers and many radiation oncologists must rely on CT and PET images obtained at separate acquisitions as described above. Modern treatment planning systems such as Focalease (Computerized Medical Systems Inc., St. Louis, Missouri) and Pinnacle (Philips Medical Systems, Eindhoven, The Netherlands) allow seamless transfer of PET/CT data into the contouring workspace and provide a wide range of options for display of fused PET and CT images. Fig. 2 shows a PET/CT scanner (Discovery LS; GE Medical Systems, Milwaukee, WI) in use at our institution, illustrating the flat couch top and laser system essential for accurate patient positioning for radiotherapy planning. Fig. 3 shows a typical screenshot of a patient who has lung cancer undergoing radiotherapy planning, using Focalsim (Computerized Medical Systems Inc.).

Delineation of metabolic/structural target volumes

The advent of PET/CT planning has opened up new challenges in planning RT. There has been little guidance from the literature on how best to use PET/CT information in contouring tumor and target volumes and there are some new technical difficulties for the radiation oncologist to consider.

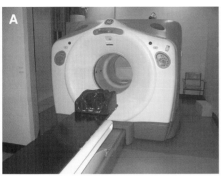
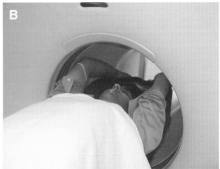

Fig. 2. (A) PET/CT scanner with flat couch top and patient-positioning device for lung cancer. (B) Positioning on PET/CT scanner for radiotherapy planning with the aid of lasers.

Some types of PET information are easy to incorporate into treatment planning. A lymph node that is negative for tumor by CT criteria but is unequivocally involved on PET can easily be incorporated into the target volume. Changes to the perceived status of the thoracic lymph node stations have the biggest influence on changing target volumes in the treatment of NSCLC. Similarly, enlarged nodes that are not metabolically active on PET may be omitted from the GTV if considered unlikely to contain tumor, and this is simple to accomplish.

In contrast, there can be a major difficulty in determining the boundaries of some tumors that do not have clearly delineated margins on CT component of PET/CT [34]. This is due to the relatively low resolution of the PET part of the image and the consequent blurriness of the edge of many structures visualized on PET scans. When the edge

of a tumor gradually merges into adjacent normal tissues, it can be difficult to decide where to place the contour that defines the edge of the lesion when determining the GTV. Motion of the patient on the couch top, which should be minimal with appropriate positioning and immobilization, and internal motion, such as that related to respiration or the cardiac cycle that can only be compensated for by gated acquisition of the PET data, also contribute to the blurriness of PET images. Other confounding factors may include regions of low avidity in the tumor due to necrosis and poor contrast between tumors with a low standardized uptake value and adjacent normal structures. Whereas CT information is acquired almost instantaneously and represents a snapshot in time, PET information is acquired over many respiratory and cardiac cycles and therefore represents an "average" position of

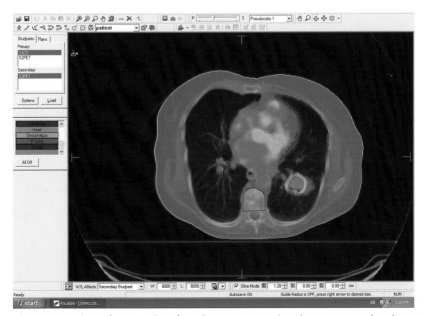

Fig. 3. Screenshot of PET/CT data for a lung cancer patient in treatment planning workstation.

the structures imaged. Tumor movement will be discussed further below.

There are two main approaches to contouring the edges of tumors on PET/CT. The first, which is preferred at our institution, is to use a standardized visual approach. At the Peter MacCallum Cancer Center (Melbourne, Australia), PET/CT data are displayed using uniform window settings and color settings. All available information is used in an "intelligent" process, including PET and CT data, biopsy reports, and the results of fluoroscopy to assess tumor movement. We have considerable institutional experience of comparing individual PET/CT scan information with surgical findings in operable cases and this experience is helpful in the planning process for unresectable tumors. The contouring of the GTV is only performed following consultation with the nuclear medicine physician who is asked to draw around the edge of the tumor on a hard copy of the PET/CT scan. Alternatively, the PET physician may be present in the radiotherapy planning area. Preliminary reproducibility studies at our center, so far unpublished, suggest that this approach gives similar results if the GTV is contoured by a radiologist, PET physician, or radiation oncologist. It must be emphasized that this approach should be used in the setting of a rigorous contouring protocol.

The second approach to contouring recognizes that visual methods can suffer from unacceptable variability due to human factors and makes use of the quantitative information available from PET. Various automated or semi-automated approaches are being tried for tumor contouring [32,35–37], but none of these methods has yet proven to be a comprehensive solution to the problem in vivo [38] although static phantoms can be effectively contoured [31]. In a clinical setting, all of the automated approaches must frequently be overridden by a human operator, because FDG uptake is not just due to malignant processes; it can also result from a range of inflammatory and physiological conditions that no computer software can recognize but often can be readily recognized by an experienced physician (eg, uptake in brown fat or muscle, sarcoidosis, and so forth). An increase in reproducibility could potentially be associated with a decrease in accuracy unless each computer-derived tumor contour is carefully analyzed and edited by the radiation oncologist, who bears final responsibility for the planning process.

Movement

The region of three-dimensional space within which a lesion moves can be referred to as the internal target volume [31,37]. This is often well appreciated on PET scanning because of the long acquisition time. Metabolic lesions are usually qualitatively enlongated in the axes of respiratory movement compared with their true dimensions, reflecting temporal blurring of activity, unless the CT image is acquired using some form of gating. Because the lesion spends relatively less time at the extremes of respiratory excursion, particularly at the end of inspiration, activity tends to be less intense in those axial planes where the tumor spends proportionally less time. The PET-determined volume thus indicates most clearly the region of space where a tumor spends the most time. Accordingly a treatment centered on the PET-determined tumor volume is likely to be aimed correctly [39,40].

Role of PET in radiation therapy planning in non–small cell lung cancer

Lung cancer is the malignancy in which PET has had the greatest impact on selection of patients for radiotherapy and on radiotherapy planning [41]. This relates both to the clarity of imaging of a metabolically active cancer in a location favorable for PET and to the high rate of incremental abnormal findings seen on PET, compared with conventional imaging [42]. There is an abundance of evidence from surgical series, with systematic clinico-pathological correlation, proving that PET is much more accurate than CT in the assessment of thoracic lymph nodes, especially when CT and PET information are combined. Dwamena and colleagues [43] reviewed English-language reports on the performance of PET (14 studies, 514 patients) and CT (29 studies, 2226 patients). They reported that FDG-PET was significantly more accurate than CT ($P < .001$). The mean sensitivity was 0.79 for PET versus 0.60 for CT. The mean specificity was 0.91 for PET versus 0.77 for CT. These data can be extrapolated to radiotherapy candidates, for whom mediastinoscopy is not usually performed if the patient clearly has unresectable disease on the basis of CT findings or is medically unfit for surgery. Due to the expectation of a relatively high prevalence of nodal involvement in patients already selected for radiotherapy as the preferred treatment option, the positive predictive value of PET findings is likely to be even higher than that for surgical series, wherein a lower prevalence of mediastinal nodal involvement would tend to decrease the apparent positive predictive value allowing for a similar specificity of PET in both situations [44].

Another crucial advantage of PET is the ability to image distant metastases and thereby exclude patients who have incurable metastatic disease from futile aggressive attempts at cure [45]. In the absence of histopathology when imaging must be relied upon for radiotherapy planning, it is clear that the most reliable imaging for NSCLC, namely PET/CT, should be given the most weight in determining whom to treat and what anatomic sites to irradiate.

PET for selection of patients with non–small cell lung cancer for radical radiation therapy

In a large prospective study at the Peter MacCallum Cancer Centre, 153 patients who had NSCLC, all of whom were suitable candidates for radical RT on the basis of clinical assessment and conventional imaging, underwent PET scanning [11]. PET data were used for patient selection for radical RT and were also used to assist with RT planning in those who remained suitable. In that study, after PET, 30% of patients were considered unsuitable for radical RT because they had distant metastases (20%) or thoracic disease too extensive for radical irradiation (10%). Patients rejected for radical RT after PET were considered suitable only for palliative therapies and had very poor survival, but the remaining patients had very good results after aggressive therapy. A comparison of a prospective PET-staged cohort treated with radical RT/chemo RT with a comparable group of patients treated similarly in a phase III trial without PET staging at the same institution, showed that PET-staged patients had significantly better survival [28]. It is likely that this was primarily an effect of superior patient selection. Patients who had apparent stage III NSCLC, on the basis of non–PET staging investigations, had a significantly higher ($P = .016$) rate of detection of distant metastasis by PET (24%) than patients who had stage II (18%) or stage I disease (7.5%), a finding in keeping with Bayesian principles given that the ultimate distant failure rate is much higher in patients who have stage III disease [46]. The superior outcomes, however, could also have reflected superior treatment delivery in those deemed still suitable for treatment with curative intent.

Studies of PET in radiotherapy planning in lung cancer

NSCLC is the malignancy in which the effect of PET on RT planning has been most intensively studied and in which PET has had the greatest impact. Despite this fact, knowledge in this area is still limited, and no convincing data have yet been published that demonstrate superior outcomes owing to incorporation of PET into RT planning beyond the effects of superior patient selection. Nevertheless, this is an area of intensive study, and all published studies indicate that target volumes determined using PET or PET/CT are often very different from those determined using CT alone. The greatest impact

arises in patients for whom PET shows different lymph node status from CT, most commonly upstaging the extent of apparent nodal disease. A significant impact is also seen in patients who have atelectasis, where the boundary between tumor and collapsed/consolidated lung can only be identified with the aid of PET [47].

A number of studies have tried to quantify the impact of PET on RT planning in NSCLC. In our earliest study, we used PET rather than PET/CT and had no ability to coregister images [11]. Despite those limitations, we found that 22 of 102 patients had a significant increase in RT target volumes to cover new sites of disease seen only on PET. In 16 patients the target volume was reduced because regions of bland atelectasis could be excluded or enlarged nodes proved not to be FDG-avid. In 1998, Nestle and colleagues [47] reported that a significant increase in the radiation field was required to cover PET-detected disease in 9% of 34 patients, but a significant decrease was seen in 26%, especially those who had atelectasis. Munley and colleagues [48] recorded that 35% of 35 patients had an increase in the RT field as a result of PET. In a larger study of 73 patients, Vanuytsel and colleagues [49] found that there was an increase in GTV in 22% of patients and a decrease in 40%. Other significant studies include work by Bradley and colleagues [50], who used coregistered sequential PET and CT scans and reported increased GTV in 46% and reduced GTV in 12%. Brianzoni and colleagues [51] reported that GTV/CTV was increased in 44% and reduced in 6% of 24 lung cancer patients planned using a dedicated PET/CT scanner. Fig. 4 illustrates the difference between a PTV obtained using CT alone and one obtained using PET/CT in a patient from our current prospective RT planning trial in NSCLC.

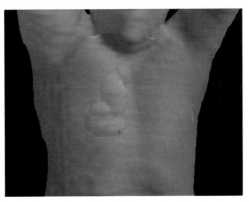

Fig. 4. Illustration of the difference in planning target volumes in a lung cancer patient obtained using CT data only (*pink*) or PET/CT (*green*). Without PET, it is likely that a geographic miss would have occurred.

Studies that did not use dedicated PET scanners for treatment planning have not been considered here because we believe that the lower sensitivity of coincidence scanners, especially for small nodes, represents a significant disadvantage compared with true PET scanning in lung cancer. Because PET-based staging is much more accurate than CT-based staging and because numerous studies have shown that radiotherapy treatment fields are significantly different if PET is used, we recommend that PET should be used in radiotherapy planning for NSCLC if it is available. Because of the very poor long-term locoregional disease control rates with RT in lung cancer [52], there is increasing interest in dose escalation of RT [53–56]. This could potentially lead to superior local control and survival but only if RT is appropriately directed. The authors believe that dose escalation without PET in many cases will be futile.

Role of PET in small cell lung cancer

Limited stage small cell lung cancer (SCLC) is potentially curable, with especially good results reported for patients treated using concurrent chemoradiation with twice daily RT fractionation. Patients who attain a complete response after primary or "induction" therapy for SCLC are at high risk for relapse with brain metastasis unless they receive prophylactic cranial irradiation. Extensive stage disease is generally considered to be incurable and is managed with chemotherapy alone. SCLC is well imaged by PET, but because it is less common than NSCLC and because treatment is often commenced soon after diagnosis because of its rapid growth rate, there are no large published series reporting the results of PET staging or restaging in this disease. At our own center, we reviewed 36 consecutive SCLC patients who underwent 47 PET studies for either staging (n = 11), restaging after therapy (n = 21), or both (n = 4). Of 15 patients who had PET for staging, 5 (33%) were upstaged from limited to extensive disease and treated without thoracic radiotherapy [57]. Twenty-five patients underwent 32 restaging PET scans, of which 20 (63%) were discordant with conventional imaging. In 8 cases, PET showed more extensive disease than conventional imaging, and in 12 cases PET-apparent disease appeared less extensive. In 13 patients, 14 untreated discordant lesions were evaluable; PET was confirmed accurate in 11 (79%) sites by last follow-up. These results are similar to those reported by other groups [58–62], suggesting that PET may have a role to play in selecting patients for RT and in designing the RT fields. PET may also be useful in defining complete remission

more accurately so that patients may be appropriately selected for PCI.

Potential for new tracers

Although FDG provides an excellent combination of sensitivity and specificity for most clinical oncological settings, it should be recognized that it simply visualizes a basic biochemical function of most living cells (ie, their ability to use glucose as an energy substrate). Lack of specificity of glucose metabolism as a target for disease detection is particularly relevant for the detection of cancer. Because enhanced glycolytic metabolism is a characteristic of many cancers but also of active inflammatory processes, cancer staging can be compromised by apparent focal accumulations of FDG due to infectious diseases, granulomatous lesions, and inflammatory healing responses related to previous interventions or therapies. Although pattern recognition can play an important role in differentiating these processes [63], biopsy may be necessary to definitively confirm the nature of FDG PET abnormalities. Even when cancer is known to be present, high uptake in adjacent tissues due to physiologic processes can reduce lesion contrast and thereby impair the sensitivity of FDG-PET for the detection of disease. The most obvious example of this is in the brain where high glucose use by the normal cortex can mask the presence of brain tumors but can also happen in lung cancer where postobstructive pneumonia can impair differentiation of NSCLC from adjacent inflammatory changes. Low FDG avidity can also occur with certain tumors and reduce contrast and, therefore, sensitivity even in the absence of high background activity. Bronchioloalveolar lung cancer is but one example of tumors of this type [64]. New tracers offer the potential to address both these limitations and also to establish new applications for PET, particularly in target disease specific clinical applications.

In an era where molecular profiling is identifying specific and mechanistically important alterations in diseased cells, a logical progression of PET tracer development is to go beyond probing of basic biochemical processes to looking at more specific features of cancer biology. With respect to radiation oncology, the concept of subpopulations of cells with differing radiosensitivity and capacity for repopulation may be important to the design of treatment schedules and dose. Rapidly proliferating tumors may have greater potential for repopulation and thereby benefit from accelerated treatment regimens, as is exemplified by the results of continuous hyperfractuioinated accelerated radiotherapy (CHART) in NSCLC [65] or head and neck cancer [66]. Alternatively, hypoxic cells often have a low proliferative fraction and are more likely to be radioresistant. Both these processes can now be imaged with PET. The cellular uptake of fluorothymidine provides evaluation of cellular proliferation and has been found to correlate with the immuno-histochemical proliferation marker ki-67 [67].

Extensive efforts have also been made to develop PET tracers to enable the noninvasive imaging of hypoxia. ^{18}F-fluoromisonidazole (FMISO) is the most extensively studied agent and has been shown to stratify prognosis in patients receiving conventional radiotherapy [27,68]. However, FMISO is a relatively lipophilic compound and demonstrates relatively low uptake in hypoxic tissue relative to normal tissue, and slow clearance from normal tissues requiring delayed scanning with consequences on contrast and image quality. This has led to the development of other hypoxic tracers with more favorable imaging properties. ^{18}F-fluoro-azomycin arabinoside (FAZA) is one such agent [69]. Preliminary results have been obtained at our institution with the use of FAZA to image hypoxia within head and neck squamous cell carcinomas. These suggest that FAZA is likely to be a superior agent for hypoxia imaging and it may have applicability in lung cancer.

^{18}F-fluoromethyl-dimethyl-2-hydroxyethyl-ammonium or fluorocholine (FCH) is also an interesting new tracer. Tumor tissues have a requirement for increased synthesis of phosphatidylcholine, an important constituent of cell membranes. Increased rates of transmembrane transport and subsequent phosphorylation of choline by the enzyme choline kinase in tumors have been demonstrated. Preliminary studies suggest that FCH may be more sensitive than FDG for detection of nodal and bone metastases in prostate cancer [70]. In defining the need and extent of radiotherapy for suspected nodal involvement in patients who have prostate cancer, FCH may prove superior to FDG because of higher sensitivity for disease detection.

Summary

PET is transforming the way radiation oncologists approach lung cancer and is contributing to increasing optimism in our approach to this group of diseases. PET has an even bigger impact on the management of patients who have lung cancer treated with radiation than on those managed with surgery. This is because of the very high rates of abnormal findings in patients who have more advanced disease and because RT candidates do not undergo comprehensive surgical staging. PET selection alone is enough to improve our apparent success rate with this modality. PET/CT therefore represents the best quality information that we can get for most patients, and it differs considerably from the information that we previously obtained from CT alone. The authors believe that we are in the early stages of a revolution in thoracic oncology, one in which PET staging will become a standard part of the evaluation of all patients who are candidates for definitive RT for lung cancer and in which PET data will be seamlessly integrated into the treatment planning process.

References

[1] Chang JY, Liu HH, Komaki R. Intensity modulated radiation therapy and proton radiotherapy for non-small cell lung cancer. Curr Oncol Rep 2005;7(4):255–9.

[2] Svensson H, Moller TR. Developments in radiotherapy. Acta Oncol 2003;42(5–6):430–42.

[3] Drzymala RE, Mohan R, Brewster L, et al. Dose-volume histograms. Int J Radiat Oncol Biol Phys 1991;21(1):71–8.

[4] Ling CC, Burman C, Chui CS, et al. Conformal radiation treatment of prostate cancer using inversely-planned intensity-modulated photon beams produced with dynamic multileaf collimation. Int J Radiat Oncol Biol Phys 1996;35(4):721–30.

[5] Leibel SA, Fuks Z, Zelefsky MJ, et al. Intensity-modulated radiotherapy. Cancer J 2002;8(2):164–76.

[6] Pickles T, Pollack A. The case for dose escalation versus adjuvant androgen deprivation therapy for intermediate risk prostate cancer. Can J Urol 2006;13(Suppl 2):68–71.

[7] Bussels B, Maes A, Hermans R, et al. Recurrences after conformal parotid-sparing radiotherapy for head and neck cancer. Radiother Oncol 2004; 72(2):119–27.

[8] Mountain CF. Lung cancer staging classification. Clin Chest Med 1993;14(1):43–53.

[9] Luciani A, Itti E, Rahmouni A, et al. Lymph node imaging: basic principles. Eur J Radiol 2006; 58(3):338–44.

[10] Webb WR, Gatsonis C, Zerhouni EA, et al. CT and MR imaging in staging non-small cell bronchogenic carcinoma: report of the Radiologic Diagnostic Oncology Group. Radiology 1991; 178(3):705–13.

[11] MacManus MP, Hicks RJ, Ball DL, et al. F-18 fluorodeoxyglucose positron emission tomography staging in radical radiotherapy candidates with nonsmall cell lung carcinoma: powerful correlation with survival and high impact on treatment. Cancer 2001;92(4):886–95.

[12] Vansteenkiste JF, Stroobants SG. Positron emission tomography in the management of non-small cell lung cancer. Hematol Oncol Clin North Am 2004;18(1):269–88.

[13] Wirth A, Seymour JF, Hicks RJ, et al. Fluorine-18 fluorodeoxyglucose positron emission tomography, gallium-67 scintigraphy, and conventional

staging for Hodgkin's disease and non-Hodgkin's lymphoma. Am J Med 2002;112(4):262–8.

[14] Jerusalem G, Beguin Y, Fassotte MF, et al. Whole-body positron emission tomography using 18F-fluorodeoxyglucose for posttreatment evaluation in Hodgkin's disease and non-Hodgkin's lymphoma has higher diagnostic and prognostic value than classical computed tomography scan imaging. Blood 1999;94(2):429–33.

[15] Pramesh CS, Mistry RC. Role of PET scan in management of oesophageal cancer. Eur J Surg Oncol 2005;31(4):449.

[16] Flamen P, Lerut A, Van Cutsem E, et al. Utility of positron emission tomography for the staging of patients with potentially operable esophageal carcinoma. J Clin Oncol 2000;18(18):3202–10.

[17] Grigsby PW, Siegel BA, Dehdashti F. Lymph node staging by positron emission tomography in patients with carcinoma of the cervix. J Clin Oncol 2001;19(17):3745–9.

[18] Follen M, Levenback CF, Iyer RB, et al. Imaging in cervical cancer. Cancer 2003;98(9 Suppl): 2028–38.

[19] Kalff V, Hicks RJ, Ware RE, et al. Evaluation of high-risk melanoma: comparison of [18F]FDG PET and high-dose 67Ga SPET. Eur J Nucl Med Mol Imaging 2002;29(4):506–15.

[20] Wagner JD. Fluorodeoxyglucose positron emission tomography for melanoma staging: refining the indications. Ann Surg Oncol 2006;13(4): 444–6.

[21] Hicks RJ, Toner GC, Choong PF. Clinical applications of molecular imaging in sarcoma evaluation. Cancer Imaging 2005;5(1):66–72.

[22] Esteves FP, Schuster DM, Halkar RK. Gastrointestinal tract malignancies and positron emission tomography: an overview. Semin Nucl Med 2006;36(2):169–81.

[23] Gyorke T, Zajic T, Lange A, et al. Impact of FDG PET for staging of Ewing sarcomas and primitive neuroectodermal tumours. Nucl Med Commun 2006;27(1):17–24.

[24] Franzius C, Schober O. Assessment of therapy response by FDG PET in pediatric patients. Q J Nucl Med 2003;47(1):41–5.

[25] Floeth FW, Pauleit D, Wittsack HJ, et al. Multimodal metabolic imaging of cerebral gliomas: positron emission tomography with [18F]fluoroethyl-L-tyrosine and magnetic resonance spectroscopy. J Neurosurg 2005;102(2):318–27.

[26] Yap CS, Czernin J, Fishbein MC, et al. Evaluation of thoracic tumors with 18F-fluorothymidine and 18F-fluorodeoxyglucose-positron emission tomography. Chest 2006;129(2):393–401.

[27] Rischin D, Hicks RJ, Fisher R, et al. Prognostic significance of [18F]-misonidazole positron emission tomography-detected tumor hypoxia in patients with advanced head and neck cancer randomly assigned to chemoradiation with or without tirapazamine: a substudy of Trans-Tasman Radiation Oncology Group Study 98.02. J Clin Oncol 2006;24(13):2098–104.

[28] MacManus MP, Wong K, Hicks RJ, et al. Early mortality after radical radiotherapy for non-small-cell lung cancer: comparison of PET-staged and conventionally staged cohorts treated at a large tertiary referral center. Int J Radiat Oncol Biol Phys 2002;52(2):351–61.

[29] Ling CC, Humm J, Larson S, et al. Towards multidimensional radiotherapy (MD-CRT): biological imaging and biological conformality. Int J Radiat Oncol Biol Phys 2000;47(3):551–60.

[30] Austin-Seymour M, Kalet I, McDonald J, et al. Three dimensional planning target volumes: a model and a software tool. Int J Radiat Oncol Biol Phys 1995;33(5):1073–80.

[31] Caldwell CB, Mah K, Skinner M, et al. Can PET provide the 3D extent of tumor motion for individualized internal target volumes? A phantom study of the limitations of CT and the promise of PET. Int J Radiat Oncol Biol Phys 2003; 55(5):1381–93.

[32] Ciernik IF, Huser M, Burger C, et al. Automated functional image-guided radiation treatment planning for rectal cancer. Int J Radiat Oncol Biol Phys 2005;62(3):893–900.

[33] Ackerly T, Andrews J, Ball D, et al. Display of positron emission tomography with Cadplan. Australas Phys Eng Sci Med 2002;25(2):67–77.

[34] Nestle U, Kremp S, Schaefer-Schuler A, et al. Comparison of different methods for delineation of 18F-FDG PET-positive tissue for target volume definition in radiotherapy of patients with non-Small cell lung cancer. J Nucl Med 2005;46(8):1342–8.

[35] Davis JB, Reiner B, Huser M, et al. Assessment of (18)F PET signals for automatic target volume definition in radiotherapy treatment planning. Radiother Oncol 2006;80(1):43–50.

[36] Drever L, Robinson DM, McEwan A, et al. A local contrast based approach to threshold segmentation for PET target volume delineation. Med Phys 2006;33(6):1583–94.

[37] Chetty IJ, Fernando S, Kessler ML, et al. Monte Carlo-based lung cancer treatment planning incorporating PET-defined target volumes. J Appl Clin Med Phys 2005;6(4):65–76.

[38] Yaremko B, Riauka T, Robinson D, et al. Thresholding in PET images of static and moving targets. Phys Med Biol 2005;50(24): 5969–82.

[39] Steenbakkers RJ, Duppen JC, Fitton I, et al. Observer variation in target volume delineation of lung cancer related to radiation oncologist-computer interaction: a 'big brother' evaluation. Radiother Oncol 2005;77(2):182–90.

[40] Jin JY, Ajlouni M, Chen Q, et al. A technique of using gated-CT images to determine internal target volume (ITV) for fractionated stereotactic lung radiotherapy. Radiother Oncol 2006; 78(2):177–84.

[41] Mac Manus MP, Hicks RJ. PET scanning in lung cancer: current status and future directions. Semin Surg Oncol 2003;21(3):149–55.

[42] Gilman MD, Aquino SL. State-of-the-art FDG-PET imaging of lung cancer. Semin Roentgenol 2005;40(2):143–53.

[43] Dwamena BA, Sonnad SS, Angobaldo JO, et al. Metastases from non-small cell lung cancer: mediastinal staging in the 1990s–meta-analytic comparison of PET and CT. Radiology 1999; 213(2):530–6.

[44] Dendukuri N, Rahme E, Belisle P, et al. Bayesian sample size determination for prevalence and diagnostic test studies in the absence of a gold standard test. Biometrics 2004;60(2):388–97.

[45] MacManus MR, Hicks R, Fisher R, et al. FDG-PET-detected extracranial metastasis in patients with non-small cell lung cancer undergoing staging for surgery or radical radiotherapy–survival correlates with metastatic disease burden. Acta Oncol 2003;42(1):48–54.

[46] MacManus MP, Hicks RJ, Matthews JP, et al. High rate of detection of unsuspected distant metastases by pet in apparent stage III non-small-cell lung cancer: implications for radical radiation therapy. Int J Radiat Oncol Biol Phys 2001; 50(2):287–93.

[47] Nestle U, Walter K, Schmidt S, et al. 18F-deoxyglucose positron emission tomography (FDG-PET) for the planning of radiotherapy in lung cancer: high impact in patients with atelectasis. Int J Radiat Oncol Biol Phys 1999;44(3):593–7.

[48] Munley MT, Marks LB, Scarfone C, et al. Multimodality nuclear medicine imaging in three-dimensional radiation treatment planning for lung cancer: challenges and prospects. Lung Cancer 1999;23(2):105–14.

[49] Vanuytsel LJ, Vansteenkiste JF, Stroobants SG, et al. The impact of (18)F-fluoro-2-deoxy-D-glucose positron emission tomography (FDG-PET) lymph node staging on the radiation treatment volumes in patients with non-small cell lung cancer. Radiother Oncol 2000;55(3):317–24.

[50] Bradley J, Thorstad WL, Mutic S, et al. Impact of FDG-PET on radiation therapy volume delineation in non-small-cell lung cancer. Int J Radiat Oncol Biol Phys 2004;59(1):78–86.

[51] Brianzoni E, Rossi G, Ancidei S, et al. Radiotherapy planning: PET/CT scanner performances in the definition of gross tumor volume and clinical target volume. Eur J Nucl Med Mol Imaging 2005;32(12):1392–9.

[52] Mac Manus MP, Hicks RJ, Matthews JP, et al. Metabolic (FDG-PET) response after radical radiotherapy/chemoradiotherapy for non-small cell lung cancer correlates with patterns of failure. Lung Cancer 2005;49(1):95–108.

[53] Chen M, Hayman JA, Ten Haken RK, et al. Long-term results of high-dose conformal radiotherapy for patients with medically inoperable T1–3N0 non-small-cell lung cancer: is low incidence of regional failure due to incidental nodal irradiation? Int J Radiat Oncol Biol Phys 2006; 64(1):120–6.

[54] Nelson C, Starkschall G, Chang JY. The potential for dose escalation in lung cancer as a result of systematically reducing margins used to generate planning target volume. Int J Radiat Oncol Biol Phys 2006;65(2):573–86.

[55] Kong FM, Ten Haken RK, Schipper MJ, et al. High-dose radiation improved local tumor control and overall survival in patients with inoperable/unresectable non-small-cell lung cancer: long-term results of a radiation dose escalation study. Int J Radiat Oncol Biol Phys 2005;63(2): 324–33.

[56] Chang DT, Zlotecki RA, Olivier KR. Re-examining the role of elective nodal irradiation: finding ways to maximize the therapeutic ratio. Am J Clin Oncol 2005;28(6):597–602.

[57] Blum R, MacManus MP, Rischin D, et al. Impact of positron emission tomography on the management of patients with small-cell lung cancer: preliminary experience. Am J Clin Oncol 2004; 27(2):164–71.

[58] Bradley JD, Dehdashti F, Mintun MA, et al. Positron emission tomography in limited-stage small-cell lung cancer: a prospective study. J Clin Oncol 2004;22(16):3248–54.

[59] Brink I, Schumacher T, Mix M, et al. Impact of [18F]FDG-PET on the primary staging of small-cell lung cancer. Eur J Nucl Med Mol Imaging 2004;31(12):1614–20.

[60] Pandit N, Gonen M, Krug L, et al. Prognostic value of [18F]FDG-PET imaging in small cell lung cancer. Eur J Nucl Med Mol Imaging 2003;30(1):78–84.

[61] Kamel EM, Zwahlen D, Wyss MT, et al. Whole-body (18)F-FDG PET improves the management of patients with small cell lung cancer. J Nucl Med 2003;44(12):1911–7.

[62] Chin R Jr, McCain TW, Miller AA, et al. Whole body FDG-PET for the evaluation and staging of small cell lung cancer: a preliminary study. Lung Cancer 2002;37(1):1–6.

[63] Hicks RJ, Mac Manus MP, Matthews JP, et al. Early FDG-PET imaging after radical radiotherapy for non-small-cell lung cancer: inflammatory changes in normal tissues correlate with tumor response and do not confound therapeutic response evaluation. Int J Radiat Oncol Biol Phys 2004;60(2):412–8.

[64] Heyneman LE, Patz EF. PET imaging in patients with bronchioloalveolar cell carcinoma. Lung Cancer 2002;38(3):261–6.

[65] Saunders M, Dische S, Barrett A, et al. Continuous hyperfractionated accelerated radiotherapy (CHART) versus conventional radiotherapy in non-small-cell lung cancer: a randomised multicentre trial. CHART Steering Committee. Lancet 1997;350(9072):161–5.

[66] Saunders MI, Dische S, Barrett A, et al. Randomised multicentre trials of CHART vs conventional radiotherapy in head and neck and non-small-cell lung cancer: an interim report.

CHART Steering Committee. Br J Cancer 1996; 73(12):1455–62.

[67] Vesselle H, Grierson J, Muzi M, et al. In vivo validation of 3'deoxy-3'-[(18)F]fluorothymidine ([(18)F]FLT) as a proliferation imaging tracer in humans: correlation of [(18)F]FLT uptake by positron emission tomography with Ki-67 immunohistochemistry and flow cytometry in human lung tumors. Clin Cancer Res 2002;8(11): 3315–23.

[68] Eschmann SM, Paulsen F, Reimold M, et al. Prognostic impact of hypoxia imaging with 18F-misonidazole PET in non-small cell lung cancer and head and neck cancer before radiotherapy. J Nucl Med 2005;46(2):253–60.

[69] Piert M, Machulla HJ, Picchio M, et al. Hypoxia-specific tumor imaging with 18F-fluoroazomycin arabinoside. J Nucl Med 2005;46(1): 106–13.

[70] DeGrado TR, Coleman RE, Wang S, et al. Synthesis and evaluation of 18F-labeled choline as an oncologic tracer for positron emission tomography: initial findings in prostate cancer. Cancer Res 2001;61(1):110–7.

POSITRON
EMISSION
TOMOGRAPHY

PET Clin 1 (2006) 329–337

Evaluation of Cost-effectiveness of FDG-PET in Non–Small Cell Lung Cancer

Otto S. Hoekstra, MD, PhD[a],*, Harm van Tinteren, MSc[b],
Egbert F. Smit, MD, PhD[c]

- [18]FDG-PET and non-small cell lung cancer
- Literature analysis
- Residual inefficiency of daily practice
- Decision-modeling
- Exploring "clinical value"
- Randomized controlled trials

- Economic evaluation
- Guideline development
- Residual inefficiency and new developments
- References

New health care technology often entails the dilemma of rapid diffusion, inspired by considerable clinical benefit versus adequate evaluation, followed by implementation in appropriate clinical situations. This has been recognized shortly after the introduction of computed tomography in 1973 [1] and later with the introduction of MR imaging [2]. Compared with therapeutic interventions, the evaluation of a diagnostic test is particularly challenging because results may be less directly linked to health outcomes.

Diagnosis and staging of cancer involves a multidisciplinary step-by-step process. The goal of that process is to determine the most likely stage of disease to give the patient the therapy that is most appropriate. Each diagnostic test contributes a piece of information. In diagnostic accuracy studies, this information is usually expressed in a two-by-two table: the test is either positive or negative, and the disease is present or absent. A series of statistics are based on these combinations. The most common accuracy measures are: (1) sensitivity, the number of true test positives divided by all cases with disease and (2) specificity, the number of true test negatives divided by all cases without the disease. In reality however, unless the test result is pathognomonic (eg, multiple bone metastases at bone scintigraphy), test results are less of a "black-and-white" condition. Recently, a radiologist who had been forced to express himself in a language that was not his own explained: "Sitting on the fence—a radiologist's stock in trade—necessitates using words for balance, weighing diagnostic probabilities, and leaning toward the heavier side. But because I couldn't use

This work was supported by a grant from the ZonMw Program, The Netherlands Organization for Health Research and Development, and the Health Care Efficiency Research Program.
[a] Department of Nuclear Medicine & PET Research, VU University Medical Center, De Boelelaan 1117, 1081 HV Amsterdam, The Netherlands
[b] Comprehensive Cancer Center Amsterdam, Plesmanlaan 125, Amsterdam, The Netherlands
[c] Department of Pulmonary Diseases, VU University Medical Center, De Boelelaan 1117, 1081 HV Amsterdam, The Netherlands
* Corresponding author.
E-mail address: os.Hoekstra@vumc.nl (O.S. Hoekstra).

doi:10.1016/j.cpet.2006.09.003

the subjunctive mood, I was forced into the realm of apparent diagnostic certainty" [3].

FDG-PET is generally evaluated visually and the nuclear medicine physician reports abnormal uptake in qualitative terms ("faint, moderate, and intense uptake"). Unfortunately, lack of standardization and validated thresholds, which account for partial volume effects, limit the use of semiquantitative measures such as the standardized uptake value. Translated into a diagnosis, the qualifications should be interpreted somewhere between definitively benign, probably benign, equivocal, probably malignant, or definitively malignant. Obviously the dichotomy is lost. Likewise, each individual (noninvasive) test adds some probability measure and usually only invasively obtained tissue material provides histological proof of disease.

When clinical decision-making is multifactorial and test results are imperfect, improved diagnostic accuracy provided by one component of a diagnostic test sequence may not necessarily translate into meaningful therapeutic changes. Obviously, without evidence of changes in therapeutic decisions, the implementation of new tests is unlikely to have impact on health or costs.

Several experts in health technology assessment advocate a hierarchical approach to the assessment of diagnostic imaging technology [4]. This stepwise framework typically is as follows:

1. Evaluation of technical and image quality and diagnostic performance (sensitivity and specificity)
2. Assessment of diagnostic and therapeutic impact
3. Measurement of effectiveness on patient and societal outcomes needs
4. Defining costs and benefits of the implementation

Although this approach has been cited and discussed frequently in the literature, neither CT nor MR imaging were assessed accordingly before clinical adoption. Typically, the first two levels were studied extensively, but the implementation of the technique happened independently of evidence from the levels that were beyond accuracy. In 2003, Jarvik and colleauges published the results of a randomized controlled trial (RCT) comparing MR imaging with plain radiographs in patients that were referred to the hospital for radiographical evaluation of low back pain [5]. Improvements in the MR imaging technique had made the comparison a clinically relevant issue. Both imaging techniques resulted in nearly identical outcomes of disability, pain, and general health status for patients. However, MR imaging increased the costs of care because of the higher costs of the technique itself and the increased number of needed operations and specialist consultations. Although physicians preferred

using MR imaging, substituting this process for radiographs in primary care of low back pain is not indicated. It is not relevant whether the negative trial outcome results from a lack of diagnostic quality or from a lack of therapeutic efficacy; the bottom line is that MR imaging should not be used in a routine setting for this problem. The level of information provided by accuracy studies can be compared with that from phase II studies in the evaluation of treatments. These studies are a prerequisite in the process of building evidence of activity, but are not suited to producing information on the difference between the effects of a new drug and those of other competing drugs or devices.

^{18}FDG-PET and non–small cell lung cancer

The following paragraphs discuss the process of evaluation and the results of clinical research on the cost-effectiveness of FDG-PET in non–small cell lung cancer (NSCLC), with an emphasis on the authors' own experience in The Netherlands.

In 1996, the VU Medical Center (VUMC) acquired a dedicated PET scanner, which was the second scanner in The Netherlands. Since the VUMC served a population of 2.5 million people, the authors anticipated a lack of scan capacity for oncological PET. Data were needed to decide for which clinical indications and at what point in the diagnostic workup ^{18}FDG-PET would be most beneficial. ^{18}FDG-PET was mostly suggested as an "add-on" technique, but it might also substitute for other diagnostic procedures. Our main concern however, was to ensure equity of access to this new technology.

The authors' PET evaluation strategy started some years before the actual installation of the PET scanner in their region, with surveys of the literature and of the residual inefficiency of prevailing daily clinical practice.

Literature analysis

When searching for evidence on the value of a diagnostic imaging technique, typically data on diagnostic accuracy dominate the literature. Aggregation of such data should be done in a systematic review. Standards for the design, execution, and reporting of accuracy studies and subsequent meta-analysis are now in place. The authors recommend applying the guidelines of the Cochrane Collaboration on reviewing techniques (www.cochrane.org), and initiatives such as the Standards for Reporting of Diagnostic Accuracy [6] and the Quality Assessment of Studies of DiagnosticAccuracy included in Systematic Reviews instrument [7] for reporting diagnostic accuracy and for assessing the quality of accuracy studies, respectively. Without promising results from accuracy studies, preferably summarized in systematic reviews, higher-level efficacy studies are not warranted.

In 1996, a comprehensive report from the Management Decision and Research Center Technology Assessment Program was published with a systematic review of the literature on [18]FDG-PET as a diagnostic test for potential applications mainly in neurology, cardiology, and oncology [8]. Motivated by positive accuracy studies, further research was suggested to define the impact of [18]FDG-PET on treatment decision-making and on outcomes in comparison with existing techniques.

Residual inefficiency of daily practice

To assess the potential benefit of a new test in clinical practice, it is necessary to have detailed knowledge of the situation before the introduction of that test. Local facilities, individual expertise, and diagnostic workup practices may vary substantially even within a relatively small geographic area. Because of such variations, potential benefit of a new device may differ between hospitals or practices. Furthermore, the observed level and nature of the (in)efficiency provides the parameters required for sample sizes and other statistical considerations of new studies. Finally, data on the regional situation will help to interpret results from other studies and to assess the generalizability. Preferably such studies are performed on patient files and electronic registries because those reveal the actual behavior. Inclusion of different types of institutes will improve external validity of the results and has the additional benefit that a committed network of investigators is formed for further research.

The authors reviewed clinical practice, yield, and costs of preoperative staging for suspected NSCLC in the medical records of all patients diagnosed between 1993 and 1995 in an academic and a large community hospital [9]. Cross-linking with the Dutch Cancer Registry and the Pathological Anatomical National Registry, complete surgical, histopathologic, and follow-up data were provided. The authors found a high adherence to international guidelines, despite practice variation between the two hospitals. Hospitals differed in the setting of diagnostic staging (hospitalization, outpatient setting) and the extent of mediastinoscopy use. The authors found that in nearly 50% of operated patients who have NSCLC, surgical treatment failed because of an irresectable tumor or a benign lesion during surgery, recurrence, or metastases within 1 year after surgery. During surgery, 33 (23% of patients who underwent surgery) were not resectable, and 19 (13%) had a benign lesion. The authors further classified surgery as futile in 18 patients (13%) who developed metastases or local

recurrence (n = 1) within 12 months following presumed curative surgery. The effort of staging proved to be considerable in terms of diagnostic load (mean of five diagnostic tests [SD ± 1.5]) conducted over a median of 20 days and in 13%, more than 6 weeks. Together with the literature survey on [18]FDG-PET, these data clearly indicated that there was room for improvement in the preoperative diagnostic process and that the nature of the problems might partially be resolved by [18]FDG-PET.

Decision-modeling

Decision analysis models the cost-effectiveness of a new diagnostic device. The model can combine results of clinical studies that cover different health care steps. In the presence of many alternative diagnostic strategies, decision analysis can help to identify the most promising diagnostic tests or algorithms for further research [10,11]. The data input is usually based on a meta-analysis of accuracy studies [11]. Unfortunately accuracy studies often fail basic quality standards (eg, independence of test interpretation, sample size, and case selection) [12,13]. In addition, decision analyses studies require a large number of assumptions to make decision problems tractable [4]. As a consequence, decision analysis is often only of limited value when faced with the complexity of daily clinical practice, as well as the need to make decisions with respect to clinically meaningful outcomes. As more information is generated by way of clinical studies, fewer assumptions are required for decision-modeling [14].

The authors used a decision-modeling approach to assess whether and how [18]FDG-PET might be cost-effective for routine use in the preoperative staging of patients who have NSCLC. With the input of the data collected in two Dutch hospitals, The authors considered three PET scenarios in a modeling approach: PET upfront in every patient suspected of having NSCLC [1], PET after standard imaging but before invasive staging [2], and PET only in patients considered operable and resectable after medical imaging and mediastinoscopy [3]. From a cost perspective, the second option was considered most promising [14]. Hospitalization was the major cost driver in these patients. The models predicted that introduction of [18]FDG-PET for all patients would lead to a substantial increase in staging costs, partially offset by a reduction in futile operations, given a certain amount of substitution of the current diagnostic workup. On the other hand, [18]FDG-PET before invasive staging would lead to a more limited increase in staging costs, offset by a lower level of substitution of other diagnostic tests. From a cost perspective, the evaluation of

PET in a strategy after preceding diagnostic imaging but before invasive staging seemed most optimal.

Exploring "clinical value"

Studies that determine therapeutic plans before and after the application of a new test are sometimes referred to as "clinical value" studies [15] or simply "before–after" studies [16]. By means of questionnaires, assessments of diagnostic probabilities, and assessments of provisional treatment, plans are made first without the information contributed by the imaging device and then again with the information [17]. In a third questionnaire the physician is asked to retrospectively grade the choice of therapy and the usefulness of this additional information in diagnostic understanding.

Credibility of such studies depends on a high-quality design. Specific clinical questions should be addressed, consecutive (unselected) patients presenting with a clinical problem should be entered, and changes in diagnostic certainty and therapeutic choices should be described in sufficient detail [16]. Even with attention to these issues, limitations of the clinical value study include discrepancies between the reported intention and actual clinical behavior, expectation bias, and limited generalizability. The clinical value design is most useful when the availability of the new technique is still limited. In the run-in phase toward more complex randomized studies, every patient subjected to the technique can be included to provide relevant information. Standardized feedback also helps learning of both clinicians and diagnosticians. Furthermore, in rare diseases and indications where RCTs are impossible, the clinical-value study may be the highest level of evidence possible.

To explore and improve our understanding of the potential clinical value of [18]FDG-PET in coin lesions and in a broader setting of preoperative diagnostic problems, The authors designed a before–after study. Such clinical value studies give information to diagnostic understanding and influences on therapeutic decision-making. Since its introduction at the VUMC in 1997, the effect of every oncological [18]FDG-PET scan was evaluated prospectively. Clinicians completed questionnaires just before, immediately after, and several months after the scan to study diagnostic understanding and management changes. In three years the records of over 600 consecutive patients were included with a response rate by the referring medical specialists of about 95%; half of those were referrals from outside the VUMC. Diagnostic understanding increased significantly in more than 70%, and management was changed to the benefit of the patients in 40% of all cases. The added value of the scan differed by indication. A subgroup was referred to the [18]FDG-PET center because of suspected NSCLC [18] with diagnostic dilemmas such as unclear radiological findings. After PET, clinicians reported an increase in diagnostic understanding in 84% and beneficial management changes in 50%, mostly cancelled surgery (35%). Appreciation of [18]FDG-PET increased over time. Studies with similar designs in Australia [19] and the Unites States [20] also reported significant management changes (67% and 61%, respectively) due to [18]FDG-PET.

If a clinical value study fails to show improved diagnostic understanding or therapeutic impact of an indication, it should be removed from the list of potential cost-effective tests, whereas promising results warrant further investigation.

Randomized controlled trials

The extent to which a patient may ultimately benefit from the addition of a new imaging technique (eg, a reduction in iatrogenic toxicity or improvement in [disease-free] survival) can only be investigated through a comparison of the full implementation of the technique added to, or in (partial) substitute of the conventional process. As only moderate benefit on patient outcome should be expected from any innovation, it is essential that both systematic and random errors are minimized. Balancing both known and unknown prognostic variables by randomly assigning patients to the new test or to the control group is the most efficient way to minimize error. RCTs also have several qualities and benefits that arise not from the act of randomization itself but from the fact that they have many features of high-quality research [21]. A written protocol provides transparency; the precalculation of a sample size often allows some exploration of patient and tumor characteristics that might be outcome-related, and direct cost comparisons are possible in a "real-life" setting.

Several aspects are of particular importance for RCTs involving diagnostic imaging. In therapeutic RCTs, the outcome is usually measured in terms of patient mortality and morbidity. However, diagnostic tests serve to allocate appropriate therapy to patients. A reasonable outcome measure for such studies is the extent to which appropriate therapy is applied, on the condition that the new test does not alter the definitions of staging and that agreement for treatment of each stage is already established. For example, there was a broad agreement among clinicians that treatment options of NSCLC patients would be clear when the diagnostic process had been completed. In addition, because [18]FDG-PET did not produce a new stage classification, a suitable (intermediate) outcome measure could be the reduction of iatrogenic morbidity, translated into unnecessary operations, rather than survival.

For many diagnostic tests, it is likely that they will first be applied as "add-on" to conventional workup. This is a relatively straightforward and safe approach. The moment of addition can be clearly defined in terms of logistics, as it is only necessary to have access to the technique within a reasonable time frame. However, for some tests the challenge is to study whether it can be applied earlier in the diagnostic process and may substitute other procedures. In such cases, endpoints could be shortening the workup period or the reduction in morbidity by obviating invasive procedures.

The strategy in the control group determines the extent of the contrast and is therefore essential for the interpretation of the results. Usually the choice is between current clinical practice and state-of-the-art procedures. Current clinical practice—carefully documented—as the control strategy will provide meaningful answers for the clinical community involved [4]. Our baseline study showed variances in clinical workup between hospitals. However, through several interdisciplinary sessions in the preparation phase of the RCT, a common diagnostic workup protocol could be agreed on.

In 1998, nine hospitals in our geographic region enrolled 188 patients suspected for potentially resectable NSCLC. These patients were randomly allocated to the conventional workup approach or to the same approach with [18]FDG-PET performed just before mediastinoscopy or thoracotomy [22]. The trial included approximately 65% of all eligible patients that were diagnosed in these institutes during that year. [18]FDG-PET–positive findings had to be confirmed by histology or excluded. In the conventional workup, group patients were managed as in our retrospective study. In the [18]FDG-PET add-on group, the number of futile thoracotomies was reduced by 50%. Those objective criteria for end points and clinical consensus about management of patients after diagnosis are important as illustrated by a second RCT of [18]FDG-PET in NSCLC [23]. In our study, "futile thoracotomy" pertained to objective criteria (benign lung lesion; pathologically proven mediastinal lymph-node involvement [stage IIIA-N2] other than minimal N2-disease, eg, intranodal involvement in a single lymph node established at mediastinal dissection; stage IIIB disease; explorative thoracotomy for any other reason; or recurrent disease or death from any cause within 1 year after randomization), whereas in the Australian trial the surgeon's decision was taken as the gold standard without validation against follow-up information (eg, early recurrence) [24].

The result of RCTs on a diagnostic test (sequence) should be seen in the context of patient management. In our area, there was clinical consensus that combined modality therapy (including neoadjuvant chemotherapy) should be given in case of locally advanced NSCLC. However, if an observational study on a diagnostic test identifies new prognostic subsets with unclear implication for therapy, an RCT should follow to evaluate the result of various interventions by subset rather than a trial to study the test itself.

The authors also explored the second-best option suggested by modeling and performed another RCT on [18]FDG-PET in NSCLC. This study addressed the question of replacing conventional workup with a [18]FDG-PET scan by comparing quality and substitution [25]. To this end, 465 patients were enrolled by 23 hospitals in The Netherlands to investigate substitutional performance of [18]FDG-PET if applied completely upfront in the diagnostic algorithm. The research question was whether application of [18]FDG-PET immediately after first presentation might simplify staging while maintaining accuracy, compared with the traditional strategy in routine clinical setting. Between 1999 and 2001, 465 patients (233 traditional workup, 232 PET) were enrolled by 22 hospitals. At first presentation, patients with a provisional diagnosis of lung cancer without overt dissemination were randomized to traditional workup according to international guidelines or early [18]FDG-PET followed by histologic or cytologic verification of lesions or imaging and follow-up. The mean (SD) number of procedures to finalize staging was equal in the traditional workup and PET arms: 7.9 (SD: 2.0) versus 7.9 (SD: 1.9); $P = .90$. Agreement between the clinical and final stage was good in both arms (Kappa 0.85 versus 0.78; $P = .07$). The costs did not differ significantly. In summary, the application of [18]FDG-PET alone (without concurrent CT scanning) up front in staging of patients who have (suspected) lung cancer carries similar overall quality (of accuracy) compared with traditional workup, but does not simplify staging. During these trials, the authors experienced that the window of opportunity for such research is limited. Our first trial included 65% of the eligible patients, but this accrual rate dropped to only 20% in the second trial. Apparently, the new technology had diffused too deeply into clinical and diagnostic practices already to allow an experimental setting.

Economic evaluation

One of the advantages of adding an economic evaluation to an RCT is the possibility of concurrent data collection, having the diagnostic test as the essential contrast. Health technology assessment offers a range of techniques for the evaluation of health care activities. The most common approach to economic evaluation in diagnostics is a cost-effectiveness analysis. In this type of analysis, outcome is expressed in natural units such as operations avoided or life years saved. Direct and indirect costs can be distinguished. Direct costs are defined as the resources related to the study intervention (eg, inpatient admission, medical procedures, surgery, pharmaceutical drugs, and laboratory tests). In economic evaluations, these costs are always taken into account. The importance of indirect costs depends on the research question and the perspective (eg, societal or payer) [26].

Several factors are specific to costing of diagnostic procedures. Diagnostic equipment is usually applied to many indications. For example, [18]FDG-PET is also applied to other oncologic and nononcologic indications. The number of [18]FDG-PET scans performed for these indications should also be taken into account in the calculation of the cost of one scan. However, when the procedure is cost-effective for a certain indication, one cannot automatically assume the total production capacity is being filled up with this indication. In theory, one would want to tailor the required capacity of diagnostic equipment to the cost-effectiveness for different indications. Another dilemma emerges when the capacity to perform the procedure is limited. This may either result in waiting lists, or, for the sake of the RCT, priority can be given resulting in unrealistically short waiting times. In such cases, indirect nonmedical costs of waiting times should also be considered in the economical evaluation.

Our RCT on add-on [18]FDG-PET provided direct data for comparison of costs in relation to diagnosis and therapy. Scenario analyses included various hospital settings, tracer accessibility, and scenarios for [18]FDG-PET scan usage [27]. The cost of PET varied between 736 and 1588 euros, depending on the (hospital) setting and the procurement of [18]FDG commercially or from onsite production. In the CWU group, 41% of the patients underwent a futile thoracotomy, whereas in the PET group, 21% of the thoracotomies were considered futile ($P = .003$). The average costs per patient were 9573 euros in the CWU group and 8284 euros in the PET group. The major cost driver was the number of hospital days related to recovery from surgery. Sensitivity analysis on the cost and accuracy of PET showed that the results were robust (ie, in favor of the PET group).

Guideline development

In 2001, a regional multidisciplinary committee developed a preliminary guideline on the use of [18]FDG-PET in NSCLC. Together with the growing availability of [18]FDG-PET in our region, this prioritization resulted in better access to [18]FDG-PET. In 2004, a national multidisciplinary committee developed evidence-based guidelines for diagnostic procedures and management in NSCLC [28]. [18]FDG-PET is recommended in patients who have clinical stage I–III that are medically fit for curative surgery after conventional workup and before invasive mediastinal staging. In case of suspected locoregional or hematogeneous metastases, verification is advised. If the primary tumor is not FDG avid, standard clinical procedures should be performed as in the pre-PET era unless the clinical pretest estimate of malignancy is also low and matches the PET result [29]. Mediastinoscopy, endobronchial ultrasound, or transesophageal ultrasound are advised if the primary tumor appears to be adjacent to the mediastinum at PET, reasoning that the spatial resolution of PET does not allow separation of neighboring metastatic mediastinal nodes from the primary tumor. Patients who have [18]FDG primary tumor without enlarged mediastinal lymph nodes at CT [10] or distant or extrathoracic metastases should proceed directly to surgery.

Residual inefficiency and new developments

Studying the situation before and after the implementation of the procedure including [18]FDG-PET closes the circle of studies evaluating the cost-effectiveness of a new diagnostic device. A full appreciation of the technique should take into account all perceptions, quality, and costs of its implementation. Data from the Regional Cancer Center Registry, where the PLUS study was active, indicated that the results have a substantial and lasting impact. Since the guidelines were implemented, the number of lung resections dropped an absolute 20% (corresponding to an estimated 50% reduction in unnecessary thoracotomies) compared with the average over the preceding 5 years.

Since the advent of the PET scanner, improvements in the concept of the scanner and other technologies have emerged. Recently the integrated or hybrid PET/CT scanner has been introduced [30]. Several studies have claimed that the "hardware"-fused whole body anatomic (CT) and functional (PET) images have superior accuracy compared with software fusion or visual fusion (side-by-side reading). A quick search in MEDLINE revealed five studies investigating the accuracy of the integrated PET/CT compared with the other devices in NSCLC staging [30–34]. All suggested improved accuracy for PET/CT compared with side-by-side reading of PET and CT or PET alone, and two also claimed changes in patient management [30,32]. However, the primary question should be concerned with the magnitude and nature of any residual inefficiency in current NSCLC staging. Even though the authors and others [35] are confident that adding the PET to standard diagnostic procedures reduces the number of futile thoracotomies, the authors know from the PLUS study that 20% of the thoracotomies were still unnecessary. To assess whether integrated PET/CT could have prevented these thoracotomies, the authors looked at these individual cases: in 9 patients, thoracotomy itself proved to be futile at the time of surgery, and in another 10 patients the disease recurred early (within 1 year). Of the former 9 patients, 2 had benign disease, 6 were upstaged, and 1 was not radically operated upon because the residual lung capacity precluded the pneumonectomy, which proved to be necessary to perform a complete resection. In 3 of these 6 upstaged patients, mediastinoscopy had not been able to confirm the presurgical suggestion of mediastinal involvement by PET. In the follow-up period, 4 patients relapsed after apparent curative surgery: 2 with bone metastases, 1 with metastases in the brain and skeleton after refusal of PET, and 1 with pulmonary metastases of melanoma (primary site unknown) that had been resected but in which disseminated disease became apparent during follow-up. Five patients died of surgery-related causes and 1 patient died of unknown cause. The authors recognize that these numbers are small and do not allow firm conclusions, but they might give some indication about the expected yield of PET/CT in the context of preventing unnecessary surgery.

Compared with PET alone, PET/CT clearly adds to the specificity of PET readings, and as a clinical spin-off, confirmatory biopsy procedures might be conducted more efficiently. In the PLUS study, lower cervical lymph nodes positive on PET proved to be a major challenge for radiologists in community hospitals. However, such failed confirmative procedure did not affect the number of futile thoracotomies, because lymph node involvement could be confirmed otherwise (albeit more invasively). We have argued that test results are not dichotomous in regard to the impact of PET/CT on sensitivity, and this is why PET/CT, even though it consists of the same PET and CT scanning technologies as in the stand-alone situations, might help to flip the coin toward higher levels of suspicion. However, if the suggestion raised by our PLUS study evaluation of residual problems after PET is correct, the authors do not expect major incremental benefits on that level. Claims about improved staging at the level of the primary tumor extension [30] obviously need confirmation given the limited resolution of PET [36]. Alternatively, the preliminary analysis suggests that the authors might have higher expectations

from alternative techniques to explore the mediastinum preoperatively. Endoesophageal and endobronchial ultrasound–guided fine needle aspiration are novel minimally invasive techniques with potential for the analysis of mediastinal lymph nodes partially complementary to mediastinoscopy, and of tumor invasion in centrally located tumors [37].

Alternatively, in the case of PET/CT, logistic factors may prevail that justify a switch to this modality, even when increments of clinical effectiveness or lower costs are unlikely or difficult to prove. The concept of staging a patient with a single scan, rather than with a battery of tests conducted over a period of time, is highly attractive from both a patient as well as a management perspective. Moreover, the perspective of reducing the PET scan time per patient should be appealing for those currently confronted with waiting lists.

Whichever methodological concerns the authors have about the evidence of superiority of PET/CT versus PET, the industrial development is such that PET/CT will be the standard of practice soon, simply because whole-body PET scanners are no longer being sold. An unsolved issue is whether PET/CT should be implemented up front in the diagnostic process or just before mediastinal evaluation. It is not economical to perform PET/CT on every patient if CT alone would eliminate a considerable number of surgical candidates by showing disseminated disease or benign primary pulmonary lesion. Decision analysis, preferably based on collected information of actual costs and scenario analyses, can help to clarify this issue. So far the authors have discussed FDG-PET in the context of surgical decision-making purely in terms of tumor-node-metastasis system staging issues. However, metabolic information obtained by FDG-PET also adds prognostic information at the biological level within clinical stages [38]. High uptake is prognostically unfavorable compared with tumors with lower uptake. Even though lack of standardized PET procedures impairs meta-analysis of individual studies, the point seems to have been made. How this information may be combined with other prognostic markers to develop strategies to improve the relatively poor outcome of patients who have resectable lung cancer remains to be shown, but it is likely that systemic therapy will be required in subsets of patients.

References

[1] Fineberg HV. Evaluation of computed tomography: achievement and challenge. AJR Am J Roentgenol 1978;1:1–4.

[2] Steinberg EP. Magnetic resonance coronary angiography—assessing an emerging technology. N Engl J Med 1993;12:879–80.

[3] Bruzzi JF. The words count—radiology and medical linguistics. N Engl J Med 2006;354(7): 665–7.

[4] Hunink MG, Krestin GP. Study design for concurrent development, assessment, and implementation of new diagnostic imaging technology. Radiology 2002;3:604–14.

[5] Jarvik JG, Hollingworth W, Martin B, et al. Rapid magnetic resonance imaging vs radiographs for patients with low back pain: a randomized controlled trial. JAMA 2003;289(21):2810–8.

[6] Bossuyt PM, Reitsma JB, Bruns DE, et al. Towards complete and accurate reporting of studies of diagnostic accuracy: the STARD initiative. Ann Intern Med 2003;138(1):40–4.

[7] Whiting P, Rutjes AW, Reitsma JB, et al. The development of QUADAS: a tool for the quality assessment of studies of diagnostic accuracy included in systematic reviews. BMC Med Res Methodol 2003;3:25.

[8] Flynn K, Adams E, Anderson D. Positron emission tomography. Boston: US Department of Veterans Affairs (VATAP); 1996. p. 170. HTA record 988699.

[9] Herder GJ, Verboom P, Smit EF, et al. Practice, efficacy and cost of staging suspected non-small cell lung cancer: a retrospective study in two Dutch hospitals. Thorax 2002;1:11–4.

[10] Gould MK, Kuschner WG, Rydzak CE, et al. Test performance of positron emission tomography and computed tomography for mediastinal staging in patients with non-small-cell lung cancer: a meta-analysis. Ann Intern Med 2003;11: 879–92.

[11] Gould MK, Sanders GD, Barnett PG, et al. Cost-effectiveness of alternative management strategies for patients with solitary pulmonary nodules. Ann Intern Med 2003;9:724–35.

[12] Gould MK, Maclean CC, Kuschner WG, et al. Accuracy of positron emission tomography for diagnosis of pulmonary nodules and mass lesions: a meta-analysis. JAMA 2001;7:914–24.

[13] Toloza EM, Harpole L, McCrory DC. Noninvasive staging of non-small cell lung cancer: a review of the current evidence. Chest 2003; 123(Suppl 1):137S–46S.

[14] Verboom P, Herder GJ, Hoekstra OS, et al. Staging of non-small-cell lung cancer and application of FDG-PET. A cost modeling approach. Int J Technol Assess Health Care 2002;3:576–85.

[15] Freedman LS. Evaluating and comparing imaging techniques: a review and classification of study designs. Br J Radiol 1987;719:1071–81.

[16] Guyatt GH, Tugwell PX, Feeny DH, et al. The role of before-after studies of therapeutic impact in the evaluation of diagnostic technologies. J Chronic Dis 1986;4:295–304.

[17] Wittenberg J, Fineberg HV, Ferrucci JT, et al. Clinical efficacy of computed body tomography, II. AJR Am J Roentgenol 1980;6:1111–20.

[18] Herder GJ, van Tinteren H, Comans EF, et al. Prospective use of serial questionnaires to evaluate the therapeutic efficacy of 18F-fluorodeoxyglucose (FDG) positron emission tomography (PET) in suspected lung cancer. Thorax 2003;1:47–51.

[19] Kalff V, Hicks RJ, MacManus MP, et al. Clinical impact of (18)F fluorodeoxyglucose positron emission tomography in patients with non-small-cell lung cancer: a prospective study. J Clin Oncol 2001;19:111–8.

[20] Hillner BE, Tunuguntla R, Fratkin M. Clinical decisions associated with positron emission tomography in a prospective cohort of patients with suspected or known cancer at one United States center. J Clin Oncol 2004;20:4147–56.

[21] Abel U, Koch A. The role of randomization in clinical studies: myths and beliefs. J Clin Epidemiol 1999;6:487–97.

[22] van Tinteren H, Hoekstra OS, Smit EF, et al. Effectiveness of positron emission tomography in the preoperative assessment of patients with suspected non-small-cell lung cancer: the PLUS multicentre randomised trial. Lancet 2002;359: 1388–93.

[23] Viney RC, Boyer MJ, King MT, et al. Randomized controlled trial of the role of positron emission tomography in the management of stage I and II non-small-cell lung cancer. J Clin Oncol 2004;12:2357–62.

[24] van Tinteren H, Smit EF, Hoekstra OS. FDG-PET in addition to conventional work-up in non-small-cell lung cancer. J Clin Oncol 2005; 23(7):1591.

[25] Herder GJ, Kramer H, Hoekstra OS, et al. Traditional versus up-front [18F] fluorodeoxyglucose-positron emission tomography staging of non-small-cell lung cancer: a Dutch cooperative randomized study. J Clin Oncol 2006;24(12): 1800–6.

[26] Drummond MF, Richardson WS, O'Brien BJ, et al. Users' guides to the medical literature. XIII. How to use an article on economic analysis of clinical practice. JAMA 1997;19:1552–7.

[27] Verboom P, van Tinteren H, Hoekstra OS, et al. Cost-effectiveness of FDG-PET in staging non-small cell lung cancer: the PLUS study. Eur J Nucl Med Mol Imaging 2003;11:1444–9.

[28] van Meerbeeck JP, Koning CC, Tjan-Heijnen VC, et al. [Guideline on 'non-small cell lung carcinoma; staging and treatment']. Ned Tijdschr Geneeskd 2005;149(2):72–7.

[29] Herder GJ, van Tinteren H, Golding RP, et al. Clinical prediction model to characterize pulmonary nodules: validation and added value of 18F-fluorodeoxyglucose positron emission tomography. Chest 2005;128(4):2490–6.

[30] Lardinois D, Weder W, Hany TF, et al. Staging of non-small-cell lung cancer with integrated positron-emission tomography and computed tomography. N Engl J Med 2003;25:2500–7.

[31] Antoch G, Stattaus J, Nemat AT, et al. Non-small cell lung cancer: dual-modality PET/CT in preoperative staging. Radiology 2003;229(2):526–33.

[32] Keidar Z, Haim N, Guralnik L, et al. PET/CT using 18F-FDG in suspected lung cancer recurrence: diagnostic value and impact on patient management. J Nucl Med 2004;45(10):1640–6.

[33] Cerfolio RJ, Ojha B, Bryant AS, et al. The accuracy of integrated PET-CT compared with dedicated pet alone for the staging of patients with nonsmall cell lung cancer. Ann Thorac Surg 2004;78(3):1017–23.

[34] Halpern BS, Schiepers C, Weber WA, et al. Presurgical staging of non-small cell lung cancer: positron emission tomography, integrated positron emission tomography/CT, and software simage fusion. Chest 2005;128(4):2289–97.

[35] Reed CE, Harpole DH, Posther KE, et al. Results of the American College of Surgeons Oncology Group Z0050 trial: the utility of positron emission tomography in staging potentially operable non-small cell lung cancer. J Thorac Cardiovasc Surg 2003;126:1943–51.

[36] Comans EF. Staging of non-small-cell lung cancer with integrated PET and CT. N Engl J Med 2003;349(12):1188–90.

[37] Annema JT, Hoekstra OS, Smit EF, et al. Towards a minimally invasive staging strategy in NSCLC: analysis of PET positive mediastinal lesions by EUS-FNA. Lung Cancer 2004; 44(1):53–60.

[38] Vansteenkiste J, Fischer BM, Dooms C, et al. Positron-emission tomography in prognostic and therapeutic assessment of lung cancer: systematic review. Lancet Oncol 2004;5(9):531–40.

ELSEVIER
SAUNDERS

POSITRON
EMISSION
TOMOGRAPHY

PET Clin 1 (2006) 339–346

Cost Effectiveness of Positron Emission Tomography for Characterizing Pulmonary Nodules

Michael K. Gould, MD, MS

- Introduction to cost-effectiveness analysis
- Methods of cost-effectiveness analysis
- Studies of the cost effectiveness of F-18 fluorodeoxyglucose- positron emission tomomgraphy for solitary pulmonary nodule diagnosis
- Summary
- References

The solitary pulmonary nodule (SPN) is a single, spherical radiographic opacity that measures between 8 mm and 30 mm in diameter and is completely surrounded by aerated lung [1,2]. There is no associated atelectasis, postobstructive pneumonia, pleural effusion, or hilar enlargement on the chest radiograph, and the patient is typically asymptomatic. Positron emission tomomgraphy (PET) with F-18 fluorodeoxyglucose (FDG) is now widely used to help distinguish benign from malignant lung nodules. In current practice, FDG imaging with dedicated PET has high sensitivity and intermediate specificity for characterizing the SPN [3]. As a diagnostic test, FDG-PET is more expensive than percutaneous needle biopsy, but much less expensive than surgical resection [4]. Accordingly, it is important to ask whether the diagnostic information provided by FDG-PET represents a good value for the health care dollar. Cost-effectiveness analysis (CEA) is a formal method that can be used to answer this question.

Below, the author first describes general principles of CEA, contrasts it with other forms of economic evaluation, and points out unique features of the methodology that challenge clinicians who

seek to critically evaluate studies of cost effectiveness. Next, the author compares and contrasts several studies that have examined the cost effectiveness of FDG-PET in patients with lung nodules, highlighting their limitations. Finally, the author interprets these studies to address the following question: under what circumstances is the use FDG-PET cost effective in the management of patients with SPN? Because little has been published about the diagnostic accuracy, clinical effectiveness or cost effectiveness of integrated PET-CT scanners in patients with lung nodules [5], this discussion will focus on the cost effectiveness of dedicated PET in these patients. Of note, all of the studies assumed that patients were surgical candidates. No studies have evaluated the cost effectiveness of FDG-PET in patients who are not candidates for surgery or other curative treatment.

Introduction to cost-effectiveness analysis

CEA is a type of economic evaluation that may be used to guide health care decision making. In CEA, alternative interventions are compared with respect to their resource use and expected clinical

VA Palo Alto Health Care System (111P), 3801 Miranda Avenue, Palo Alto, CA 94304, USA
E-mail address: gould@stanford.edu

doi:10.1016/j.cpet.2006.10.001

outcomes [6]. CEA is primarily concerned with efficiency, and thereby provides clinicians and policy makers with information about the relative value of an intervention. However, when making decisions regarding resource allocation, policy makers must also consider other factors, such as equity, budgetary constraints, concerns of interest groups, statutory and regulatory issues and needs for competing programs.

CEA is the type of economic evaluation that is most commonly used in health care. Other types of economic evaluations include the following [7].

A *cost analysis* compares costs for two or more interventions; health outcomes are not considered.

A *cost-minimization study* compares costs for two or more interventions; health outcomes are assumed to be equal.

A *cost-benefit analysis* compares costs and health outcomes for two or more interventions; all of the outcomes are expressed in monetary units, including the value of health and disease. This methodology is not often used in health care because some analysts and policy makers (and many physicians and patients) are uncomfortable with the idea of quantifying the economic "value of a life," although economists have developed a variety of methods to determine what a life is worth economically [8,9].

In CEA, results are typically expressed in terms of costs per life-year gained, or quality-adjusted life-year (QALY) gained. Thus, the analyst is not required to decide what a life-year or QALY is worth. Instead, the policy maker or other decision maker is left to judge whether the intervention represents a good value for the health care dollar. Therefore, CEA makes implicit what cost-benefit analysis makes explicit, and shifts the responsibility for deciding what a life is worth from the analyst to the decision maker.

A *cost-utility analysis* is a special type of CEA, in which health outcomes are expressed in terms of quality-adjusted life expectancy. In this methodology, life expectancy is weighted by "quality of life," by using a measure known as utilities. In the health care context, a utility is an individual's preference for a health state, measured under conditions of uncertainty. Utilities are grounded in the economic theory of expected value decision making, and can be considered a global measure of quality of life [10,11], although utilities are fundamentally different from psychometrically based, descriptive measures of quality of life.

Methods of cost-effectiveness analysis

There are two main ways to perform a CEA. One approach is to "piggyback" an economic evaluation alongside a conventional randomized clinical trial.

In this approach, resource use is measured prospectively, and costs (not billed charges) are assigned for each resource consumed. Thus, the short-term costs and health outcomes of two or more interventions can be compared. This approach has several advantages. First and foremost, such studies have all of the benefits of randomized trials, which are the "gold standard" for evaluating health care interventions. Second, resource use is directly measured, rather than inferred. Finally, statistical methods have been developed to determine confidence intervals for cost-effectiveness ratios [12]. The piggyback approach has several disadvantages, however. Most important, the time horizon of the analysis is limited to the duration of the clinical trial. If an expensive intervention has health benefits that continue after the end of the trial, then its cost effectiveness will be underestimated if the time horizon only includes the trial period. Another problem is that the results of this type of study may or may not be generalizable to other patient populations. In addition, such studies are expensive and difficult to perform.

More commonly, a modeling approach is used to perform CEA. Such an approach has several advantages over the piggyback method. First, modeling can be used to extend the time horizon of the analysis to cover the entire remaining life span of the patient population. The time horizon of an analysis is especially important when the intervention is designed to modify the course of a chronic disease. For example, in the economic analysis performed by the investigators of the National Emphysema Treatment Trial, lung volume reduction surgery cost $190,000 per QALY gained when a 3-year time horizon was employed, but the cost was much lower ($53,000 per QALY gained) when the authors used modeling to extend the time horizon beyond the 3-year duration of prospective data collection to 10 years [13]. This is one unique aspect of CEA that readers do not have to worry about when critically appraising other published clinical research.

Second, this approach uses data from a variety of clinical and administrative sources, which (arguably) may improve the generalizability of the findings. However, the validity of the study may be compromised if the data sources are not compatible or if the data does not fit the assumptions of the analysis, for example, if Medicare cost data is used to value outcomes for a pediatric patient population. Common sources of effectiveness data for a modeling study include results from randomized controlled trials, meta-analyses, observational studies, administrative data, and registries. Estimates of resource use can be obtained from similar sources. Costs for resources can be assigned by using proprietary cost accounting symptoms or administrative data sources, such as Medicare claims files. In general, billed charges are not an appropriate surrogate for the true opportunity cost of the resource, although methods exist for converting bundled charges to costs in some situations.

Third, the assumptions of the model can be varied in a procedure known as sensitivity analysis. Sensitivity analysis can be used to address uncertainty regarding probabilities of clinical outcomes and costs of care. Sensitivity analysis is an important way to test the robustness of the findings of a CEA, because there is always some uncertainty surrounding the many assumptions that the analyst must make. As with other research methods, CEA is a powerful tool that can be used productively or abused. The validity of a CEA is largely determined by the reasonableness of its assumptions.

Regardless of the approach, three critical questions must be asked by the reader of a CEA. What is the question? What are the alternatives? Who is the decision maker and what is his/her perspective? As is true for any other clinical research method, the research question should be clearly stated and the competing alternatives should be completely described. In addition, the intervention should be compared with the most effective alternative intervention available. Using a less effective alternative will lead to an inappropriately favorable estimate of cost effectiveness. This is particularly important when comparing three or more interventions; the cost-effectiveness ratio will be underestimated if the most effective intervention is compared with the least effective intervention instead of the next most effective alternative. To illustrate this, Fig. 1 shows that the comparison of intervention "C" with intervention "A" results in a cost-effectiveness ratio that is an order of magnitude lower than the cost-effectiveness ratio for the appropriate comparison between interventions "C" and "B."

Unlike other methods of clinical research, the issue of perspective is fundamentally important in CEA. Most published cost-effectiveness studies are structured from the "societal" perspective, which means that all costs are included, regardless of who bears them. Such a perspective is most appropriate for policy-level decision making. It is important not to generalize from one perspective to another. An intervention that represents a good value for society does not necessarily represent a good value to the health plan or individual patient. For example, when viewed from the societal perspective, outpatient treatment with low molecular weight heparin (LMWH) avoids hospitalization and saves almost $2,000 per patient treated. But when the analysis is structured from the perspective of an uninsured patient without prescription drug coverage, outpatient LMWH treatment results in out-of-pocket costs of approximately $900 [14]. This does not necessarily represent a good value for the typical uninsured patient.

Fortunately, most analyses can be structured from one or more different perspectives, including that of the patient, hospital, hospital department, or health plan, as well as that of society. The Panel on Cost Effectiveness in Health and Medicine recommends that all studies include a "reference case" analysis structured from the societal perspective, in an attempt to standardize methodology and permit comparison of results across different health care interventions [15]. Most importantly, the perspective of the analysis should be aligned with the needs of the decision maker, and the ability to generalize from one perspective to another cannot be taken for granted.

Interpreting the results of a CEA can be confusing, in part because the terminology is unfamiliar to most clinicians. By definition, a "dominant" or "cost-saving" intervention is one that is more effective and less expensive than the alternative; in such cases, the alternative intervention is said to be "dominated." Unfortunately, effective new health care interventions are typically more expensive than existing alternatives. When the expense is judged by the decision maker to be a good value, the intervention can be described as "cost effective." There is no universally accepted threshold for cost effectiveness, although some argue that societal willingness to pay for improvements in health is approximately $30,000 to $50,000 per QALY gained, because several widely accepted health care interventions have cost-effectiveness ratios that fall in this range, for example, hemodialysis for patients with end-stage renal disease, or treatment of moderate hypertension in a 60-year-old man [16].

The results of a CEA are expressed in terms of an incremental cost-effectiveness ratio, which is

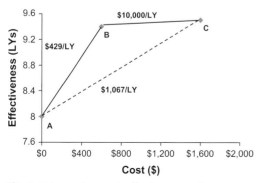

Fig. 1. Intervention cost-effectiveness ratios.

defined as the difference in costs divided by the difference in effectiveness, or:

Incremental cost-effectiveness ratio =

$$\left(\text{Cost}_{\text{Exp}} - \text{Cost}_{\text{Con}}\right) / \left(\text{Eff}_{\text{Exp}} - \text{Eff}_{\text{Con}}\right);$$

where Cost_{Exp} represents total costs associated with the experimental intervention, Cost_{Con} represents total costs associated with the next best alternative intervention, Eff_{Exp} represents the health effects in the group that received the experimental intervention, and Eff_{Con} represents the health effects in the group that received the next best alternative intervention.

In theory, the denominator of the cost-effectiveness ratio can be expressed in terms of any natural unit, for example, cases of pneumonia prevented, or the number of correct diagnoses. However, the preferred denominator for the "reference case" analysis is the QALY, because this unit captures both longevity and the quality of life, and facilitates comparison of cost effectiveness across interventions.

In summary, CEA is the most widely used type of economic evaluation in health care. Although some studies collect information about clinical effectiveness and resource use prospectively, most studies will employ modeling to extend the time horizon of the analysis and permit sensitivity analysis. Although the methods of CEA may be unfamiliar to many clinicians, a published CEA should satisfy at least the following criteria: (1) provide a comprehensive description of competing alternatives; (2) provide sufficient evidence of clinical effectiveness; (3) identify, measure, and value costs appropriately; and (4) perform sensitivity analysis to explore uncertainties [17]. In addition, the perspective and time horizon of the analysis should be clearly stated, and interventions should be compared with the next most effective alternative so that estimates of cost effectiveness are not overstated.

Studies of the cost effectiveness of F-18 fluorodeoxyglucose- positron emission tomomgraphy for solitary pulmonary nodule diagnosis

The author searched the MEDLINE database from 1966 to June 2006, by using the exploded MeSH terms "cost-benefit analysis," "tomography, emission computed," "positron-emission tomography," "lung neoplasms," "coin lesion, pulmonary," and "neoplasm staging," and identified 62 studies that were potentially relevant to the cost effectiveness of FDG-PET in patients with SPN. A careful review of titles and abstracts excluded all but eight studies. Most of the excluded studies were either review articles or studies that examined the cost effectiveness of FDG-PET for lung cancer staging. A few excluded studies evaluated PET imaging with other tracers. Two relevant studies that were from the United States will be the primary focus of this review [4,18]. Highlights of studies performed in Germany [19], Japan [20,21], Australia [22], Italy [23], and France [24] will also be discussed.

In the first US study, Gambhir and colleagues [18] used a decision analysis model to examine the cost effectiveness of four management strategies for patients with SPN. Their base-case analysis examined a 64-year-old White man with a 2.5-cm nodule on chest radiography, a 1.5 pack per day smoking history, and a life expectancy of 14.8 years (in the absence of malignancy). The four management strategies included: (1) watchful waiting with serial chest radiographs; (2) immediate surgery; (3) a strategy that began with CT, followed by watchful waiting when the CT results were "negative," and by surgery or transthoracic needle aspiration (TTNA) when CT results were "positive or indeterminate"; and (4) a strategy that employed FDG-PET selectively when CT results were "positive or indeterminate." In this strategy, the authors assumed that positive results on FDG-PET would be followed by biopsy in 20% of cases and surgery in 80% of cases, and that negative results on FDG-PET could be followed by either biopsy or watchful waiting. Although the perspective of the analysis was not clearly stated, it can be inferred that the perspective was that of the health plan, because indirect costs such as lost time from work were not included. The time horizon covered the entire lifetime for health effects, but was limited to the initial period of diagnosis and treatment for costs.

Estimates of accuracy and complication rates for imaging tests and procedures were taken from a literature review, and Medicare reimbursement rates were used to value resources that were consumed. Costs for treatment of nonmalignant disease and nonsurgical treatment of unresectable cancer were not included. Life expectancy for patients with benign nodules was assumed to be normal for age, and life expectancy for patients with malignant nodules was calculated by assuming a constant mortality rate that varied depending on the size of the nodule. This enabled the authors to estimate the reduction in mortality related to inappropriate watchful waiting in patients with malignant nodules. Although watchful waiting is widely applied in clinical practice, the risks associated with this strategy are not known. Specifically, patients with malignant nodules who are managed by watchful waiting will experience delays in diagnosis and treatment. This period of delay may result in missed opportunities for surgical cure if the cancer progresses from local to advanced stage disease. In the base-case analysis, life expectancy was assumed to be 6.6 years in patients with malignant nodules that were promptly resected, and 5.7 years in patients with malignant nodules that were resected after a period of delay lasting one tumor volume doubling time. Similar assumptions about the reduction in life expectancy due to delayed diagnosis and treatment were made by Cummings and colleagues [25] in their seminal decision analysis that compared the effectiveness of surgery, biopsy, and watchful waiting for patients with SPN. However, little or no empirical data exist to validate this assumption.

Gahmbir and colleagues [18] expressed their results in terms of incremental costs and life expectancy, without adjustment for quality of life. The patient in the base-case analysis had a calculated pretest probability of malignancy of 83%. Not surprisingly, at this (very high) probability of cancer, both the selective FDG-PET and the CT-alone strategy were much more effective than watchful waiting, and the CT-alone strategy was slightly more effective (by 0.03 years) and less expensive (by almost $400) than the selective FDG-PET strategy. Thus, in the base-case analysis, the CT alone strategy dominated the selective FDG-PET strategy, and cost only $3300 per life year gained relative to watchful waiting. Base-case results for the immediate surgery strategy were not reported.

Like Cummings and colleagues [25], they found that the choice of strategy depended critically on the pretest probability of cancer. In an initial analysis that looked at life expectancy but not costs, the choice between surgery, CT, and selective FDG-PET was a close call. Watchful waiting was preferred when pretest probability was less than 2%, the selective FDG-PET strategy was preferred when pretest probability was 2% to 44%, the CT strategy was preferred when pretest probability was 45% to approximately 80%, and surgery was preferred when the probability of cancer was greater than 80%.

When costs were included, watchful waiting was preferred when pretest probability was less than 12%, selective FDG-PET was preferred when pretest probability was 12% to 69%, CT alone was preferred when pretest probability was 70% to 90%, and surgery was preferred when the probability of cancer was greater than 90%. In this analysis, preferred strategies were defined as ones that cost less than $50,000 per QALY gained compared with watchful waiting. Because the authors did not compare strategies with the next most effective alternative at any given pretest probability, the reported cost-effectiveness ratios are difficult to interpret. For example, in the base-case analysis, they reported that the selective FDG-PET strategy had a very favorable incremental cost-effectiveness ratio of $4300

per life-year gained relative to watchful waiting; but they did not point out that selective FDG-PET was dominated by the CT-alone strategy, which was more effective and less expensive. In addition, they evaluated a limited number of possible management strategies, and did not address the question of what should be done once the results of FDG-PET are known.

More recently, Gould and colleagues [4] also used decision analysis to quantify the health effects and economic costs associated with various strategies for managing patients with pulmonary nodules. The target population for this analysis included all adult patients found to have a new, noncalcified SPN on chest radiography, no known extrathoracic malignancy, and no absolute contraindication to needle biopsy or surgical resection. The base-case analysis considered a hypothetic cohort of 62-year-old men and women, and the analysis was performed from the societal perspective, with a time horizon that covered the entire life span of the cohort. The model compared 40 clinically plausible combinations of five diagnostic interventions, including chest CT, FDG-PET imaging, TTNA, surgical resection, and watchful waiting with serial imaging. The authors performed separate analyses for patients with low (26%), intermediate (55%), and high (79%) pretest probabilities of malignancy. To estimate pretest probability, they used a model that was developed in 629 men and women with newly discovered pulmonary nodules at the Mayo Clinic and subsequently validated in a European cohort [26,27].

Gould and colleagues [4] used meta-analytic methods to estimate the diagnostic accuracy of CT, FDG-PET, and needle biopsy. To estimate long-term outcomes and costs for patients with malignant and benign pulmonary nodules, they developed a Markov model. Markov (state transition) models are often used in decision analysis to capture changes in health status over time. A simple hypothetical Markov model might contain three health states: healthy, sick, and dead. Over time, patients may transition from healthy to sick, from sick back to healthy, from sick to dead, or from healthy to dead. The analyst assigns probabilities for each health state transition over a specified period of time.

To estimate the monthly probability of cancer recurrence after surgical treatment for patients with malignant nodules, they used survival data from the Surveillance, Epidemiology, and End Results (SEER) tumor registry. To estimate monthly health care costs for patients with local, regional and distant stage lung cancer, they used data from SEER linked with Medicare claims files [28]. They used values from the literature to estimate health state utilities (quality-of-life adjustments) for patients with local, regional, and distant-stage lung cancer, and assumed that the utility of watchful waiting was normal for sex and age. To estimate the monthly probability of disease progression in patients with malignant nodules who were managed by watchful waiting, they adapted a mathematical model of the natural history of lung cancer [29–31]. They assumed that the risk of disease progression during watchful waiting depended on the growth rate of the nodule, expressed in terms of the tumor volume doubling time.

This study confirmed that the effectiveness and cost effectiveness of management strategies for patients with SPN depend critically on the pretest probability of malignancy, as well as several additional factors, including the risk of surgical complications, the probability of nondiagnostic biopsy, the sensitivity of chest CT and patient preferences for time spent in watchful waiting. Thus, it is not appropriate to adopt a "one-size-fits-all" approach to management.

The authors also found that while nonselective use of FDG-PET was highly effective for pulmonary nodule diagnosis, it was most cost effective to employ FDG-PET selectively, typically when pretest probability and CT results disagreed. For example, in patients with low pretest probability, two strategies that used FDG-PET selectively cost less than $50,000 per QALY gained under base-case model assumptions. In both of these strategies, CT was performed as the initial test, and FDG-PET was used when CT results were indeterminate (possibly malignant). Surgery was recommended when the results of FDG-PET were positive, and needle biopsy was recommended when FDG-PET results were negative. A strategy that used PET imaging nonselectively was marginally more effective, but cost nearly $300,000 per QALY gained.

In patients with intermediate pretest probability (55%), PET strategies cost more than $200,000 per QALY gained, because they were considerably more costly, but only marginally more effective than strategies that did not include PET. In these patients, three strategies that used CT without FDG-PET cost less than $20,000 per QALY gained. In the most effective of these strategies, surgery was performed when CT results were indeterminate (possibly malignant) and needle biopsy was performed when CT results were benign.

Several other variables affected the choice of strategy, including the probability of nondiagnostic needle biopsy in patients with malignant nodules and patient preferences regarding watchful waiting. Selective use of FDG-PET was economically attractive in patients with intermediate pretest probability when we assumed that the probability of nondiagnostic biopsy was twice as high as the base-case value (17% versus 9%), and when the relative utility of the time spent in observation was assumed to be 0.97 or less (base-case value 1.00). A relative utility of 0.97 implies that an individual would accept a 3% risk of instant death to know whether the nodule was malignant or benign.

Despite widely differing assumptions across models, a sensitivity analysis on pretest probability identified similar thresholds as Cummings and colleagues [25] and Gambhir and colleagues [18]. Specifically, watchful waiting was preferred when the probability of malignancy was less than 3%, TTNA was preferred when the probability of malignancy was 3% to 20%, FDG-PET was preferred when the probability of malignancy was 21% to 72%, and surgery was preferred when the probability of cancer was >72%. In this analysis, a preferred strategy was defined as one that was most effective and cost less than $100,000 per QALY gained.

The most important limitation of this study is that there is no way to empirically validate the authors' estimate of reduced life expectancy in patients with malignant nodules who undergo watchful waiting. The natural history model indicated that delaying diagnosis and treatment by one tumor volume doubling time would reduce life expectancy by almost 30%. However, results of the CEA were similar when they used the more conservative estimates of reduced life expectancy (~14%) that were assumed by Gambhir and colleagues [18]. In addition, the model did not capture other potential benefits of FDG-PET, such as the ability to identify occult regional or distant metastases, although these are relatively uncommon in patients with T1 tumors [32]. Likewise, the model did not capture the potential benefit of false positive results of FDG-PET in patients with SPN caused by active infectious or inflammatory disease. Finally, some management strategies (eg, selective use of FDG-PET only after nondiagnostic results on TTNA) and possible interventions (eg, CT with dynamic contrast enhancement) were not evaluated.

The latter limitation was partly addressed by Comber and colleagues [22] in Australia, who performed a "cost-accuracy study." They modified the model used by Gambhir and colleagues [18] to compare conventional CT alone, conventional CT followed by CT with dynamic contrast enhancement (QCET), conventional CT followed by FDG-PET, and conventional CT followed by QCET and FDG-PET. A limitation of the analysis is that they compared all four strategies with a "hypothetic baseline strategy comprising no investigation or treatment." Using cost estimates from the Australian Medicare Benefits Schedule, they found that the QCET strategy had the lowest cost, and that the conventional CT strategy had the highest cost, because it results in many unnecessary biopsies and resections. The FDG-PET strategy and the FDG-PET plus QCET strategy had the highest accuracy, that is, they correctly classified the most patients with benign or malignant SPN. Based on data provided in Table 2 of the manuscript, the conventional CT strategy was dominated by the QCET strategy, and the FDG-PET strategy was dominated by the FDG-PET plus QCET strategy. Compared with the QCET strategy, the FDG-PET plus QCET strategy cost $7000 for each additional percentage increase in diagnostic accuracy. A major limitation of this study is that the measure of effectiveness (diagnostic accuracy) does not capture the different consequences of false positive and false negative test results or complications related to tests and procedures. In addition, it is difficult to interpret the results by deciding what constitutes a reasonable "cost per increase in accuracy" in the absence of well-defined benchmarks.

Another limitation was addressed by Dietlein and coworkers [19], who compared a PET-based strategy with surgery, watchful waiting, and needle biopsy. In this model, patients who had negative results on FDG-PET underwent watchful waiting; patients who had positive results in the nodule and negative results in the mediastinum underwent surgery; and patients who had positive results in the nodule and abnormal uptake in the mediastinum underwent mediastinoscopy to confirm or exclude regional metastasis. The FDG-PET strategy (which captured the ability of FDG-PET to identify occult regional lymph node metastasis) was preferred over a wide range of pretest probabilities from 5% to 75%. However, these thresholds were similar to the ones reported by Gambhir and colleagues [18] and Gould and colleagues [4]. It could also be argued that including selective or routine mediastinoscopy in the surgery strategy might have increased the effectiveness and reduced the cost of this alternative.

Summary

CEA is a formal method for quantifying the health benefits and economic costs of health care technologies. In an era when health care resources are limited, a number of Western governments have embraced CEA as a method to guide decisions about resource allocation. Because health care costs continue to increase in this country, payers will likely require evidence of cost effectiveness when making coverage decisions at some point in the future.

In recent years, multiple studies have evaluated the cost effectiveness of FDG-PET for SPN characterization, and despite using different methods and making widely different modeling assumptions, there is remarkable agreement across studies. All of the studies addressed an important clinical question: under what circumstances is the use of FDG-PET cost effective for managing patients with SPN? The answer seems to be that FDG-PET is most cost effective when used in patients with low to moderate pretest probability and indeterminate nodules on CT. In patients with indeterminate nodules and a high probability of malignancy, FDG-PET is less helpful, because a negative test result does not conclusively rule out the presence of malignancy. However, there is evidence that survival is excellent in patients with malignant nodules (T1 N0 M0 lung cancer) who have negative FDG-PET results, even when surgical resection is delayed by over 250 days [33,34]. None of the published cost-effectiveness models incorporated this information, and doing so would improve the cost effectiveness of FDG-PET-based strategies. Although the model by Gould and colleagues [4] showed that needle biopsy was slightly more effective (and marginally more expensive) than watchful waiting in patients with negative results on FDG-PET, the excellent survival in patients with PET-negative lesions supports the idea that these patients can be managed by watchful waiting in many cases. When FDG-PET results are positive, Gould and colleagues [4] showed that surgery was slightly more effective (and marginally more expensive) than needle biopsy, so PET appears to obviate the need for confirmatory biopsy before surgery. Because differences in efficacy across strategies are usually relatively small, the risks and rewards of various management alternatives should be discussed, so that the patient can make an informed decision that is consistent with his or her values and preferences.

References

[1] Ost D, Fein AM, Feinsilver SH. Clinical practice. The solitary pulmonary nodule. N Engl J Med 2003;348(25):2535–42.

[2] Tan BB, Flaherty KR, Kazerooni EA, et al. The solitary pulmonary nodule. Chest 2003;123 (1 Suppl):89S–96S.

[3] Gould MK, Maclean CC, Kuschner WG, et al. Accuracy of positron emission tomography for diagnosis of pulmonary nodules and mass lesions: a meta-analysis. JAMA 2001;285(7):914–24.

[4] Gould MK, Sanders GD, Barnett PG, et al. Cost-effectiveness of alternative management strategies for patients with solitary pulmonary nodules. Ann Intern Med 2003;138(9):724–35.

[5] Lardinois D, Weder W, Hany TF, et al. Staging of non-small-cell lung cancer with integrated

positron-emission tomography and computed tomography. N Engl J Med 2003;348:2500–7.

[6] Drummond MF, Richardson WS, O'Brien BJ, et al. Users' guides to the medical literature. XIII. How to use an article on economic analysis of clinical practice. A. Are the results of the study valid? Evidence-Based Medicine Working Group. JAMA 1997;277(19):1552–7.

[7] Cook DJ, Ellrodt AG. Systematic reviews, economic evaluations, and practice guidelines: can research synthesis help us care for the critically ill? New Horiz 1996;4(4):551–7.

[8] Landefeld JS, Seskin EP. The economic value of life: linking theory to practice. Am J Public Health 1982;72:555–66.

[9] Thompson MS. Willingness to pay and accept risks to cure chronic disease. Am J Public Health 1986;76(4):392–6.

[10] Naglie G, Krahn MD, Naimark D, et al. Primer on medical decision analysis: part 3—estimating probabilities and utilities. Med Decis Making 1997;17(2):136–41.

[11] Redelmeier DA, Detsky AS. A clinician's guide to utility measurement. Prim Care 1995;22(2):271–80.

[12] Polsky D, Glick HA, Willke R, et al. Confidence intervals for cost-effectiveness ratios: a comparison of four methods. Health Econ 1997;6(3):243–52.

[13] National Emphysema Treatment Trial Group. Cost-effectiveness of lung-volume-reduction surgery for patients with severe emphysema. N Engl J Med 2003;348(21):2092–102.

[14] Gould MK, Dembitzer AD, Sanders GD, et al. Low-molecular-weight heparins compared with unfractionated heparin for treatment of acute deep venous thrombosis: a cost-effectiveness analysis. Ann Intern Med 1999;130:789–99.

[15] Gold MR, Siegel JE, Russell LB, et al, editors. Cost-effectiveness in health and medicine. New York: Oxford University Press; 1996.

[16] Tengs TO, Adams ME, Pliskin JS, et al. Five-hundred life-saving interventions and their cost-effectiveness. Risk Anal 1995;15(3):369–90.

[17] Heyland DK, Kernerman P, Gafni A, et al. Economic evaluations in the critical care literature: do they help us improve the efficiency of our unit? Crit Care Med 1996;24(9):1591–8.

[18] Gambhir SS, Shepherd JE, Shah BD, et al. Analytical decision model for the cost-effective management of solitary pulmonary nodules. J Clin Oncol 1998;16:2113–25.

[19] Dietlein M, Weber K, Gandjour A, et al. Cost-effectiveness of FDG-PET for the management of solitary pulmonary nodules: a decision analysis based on cost reimbursement in Germany. Eur J Nucl Med 2000;27(10):1441–56.

[20] Kosuda S, Ichihara K, Watanabe M, et al. Decision-tree sensitivity analysis for cost-effectiveness of chest 2-fluoro-2-D-[(18)F]fluorodeoxyglucose positron emission tomography in patients with pulmonary nodules (non-small cell lung carcinoma) in Japan. Chest 2000;117(2):346–53.

[21] Tsushima Y, Endo K. Analysis models to assess cost-effecctiveness of the four strategies for the work-up of solitary pulmonary nodules. Med Sci Monit 2004;10(5):MT65–72.

[22] Comber LA, Keith CJ, Griffiths M, et al. Solitary pulmonary nodules: impact of quantitative contrast-enhanced CT on the cost-effectiveness of FDG-PET. Clin Radiol 2003;58(9):706–11.

[23] Gugiatti A, Grimaldi A, Rossetti C, et al. Economic analyses on the use of positron emission tomography for the work-up of solitary pulmonary nodules and for staging patients with non-small-cell-lung-cancer in Italy. Q J Nucl Med Mol Imaging 2004;48(1):49–61.

[24] Lejeune C, Bismuth MJ, Conroy T, et al. Use of a decision analysis model to assess the cost-effectiveness of 18F-FDG PET in the management of metachronous liver metastases of colorectal cancer. J Nucl Med 2005;46(12):2020–8.

[25] Cummings SR, Lillington GA, Richard RJ. Managing solitary pulmonary nodules. The choice of strategy is a "close call." Am Rev Respir Dis 1986;134(3):453–60.

[26] Swensen SJ, Silverstein MD, Ilstrup DM, et al. The probability of malignancy in solitary pulmonary nodules. Application to small radiologically indeterminate nodules. Arch Intern Med 1997;157(8):849–55.

[27] Herder GJ, van Tinteren H, Golding RP, et al. Clinical prediction model to characterize pulmonary nodules: validation and added value of 18-F-fluorodeoxyglucose positron emission tomography. Chest 2005;128:2490–6.

[28] Potosky AL, Riley GF, Lubitz JD, et al. Potential for cancer related health services research using a linked Medicare-tumor registry database. Med Care 1993;31(8):732–48.

[29] Brown BW, Atkinson EN, Bartoszynski R, et al. Estimation of human tumor growth rate from distribution of tumor size at detection. J Natl Cancer Inst 1984;72:31–8.

[30] Collins VP, Loeffler RK, Tivey H. Observations on growth rates of human tumors. Am J Roentgenol 1956;76(5):988–1000.

[31] Geddes DM. The natural history of lung cancer: a review based on rates of tumor growth. Br J Dis Chest 1979;73:1–17.

[32] Seely JM, Mayo JR, Miller RR, et al. T1 lung cancer: prevalence of mediastinal nodal metastases and diagnostic accuracy of CT. Radiology 1993;186(1):129–32.

[33] Cheran SK, Nielsen ND, Patz EF Jr. False-negative findings for primary lung tumors on FDG positron emission tomography: staging and prognostic implications. AJR Am J Roentgenol 2004;182(5):1129–32.

[34] Marom EM, Sarvis S, Herndon JE 2nd, et al. T1 lung cancers: sensitivity of diagnosis with fluorodeoxyglucose PET. Radiology 2002;223(2):453–9.

POSITRON
EMISSION
TOMOGRAPHY

PET Clin 1 (2006) 347–352

PET Versus PET/CT Dual-Modality Imaging in Evaluation of Lung Cancer

Lutz S. Freudenberg, MD, MA, MBA[a],*, Sandra J. Rosenbaum, MD[a],
Thomas Beyer, PhD[a], Andreas Bockisch, PhD, MD[a],
Gerald Antoch, MD[b]

- FDG-PET/CT versus FDG-PET
- FDG-PET/CT versus FDG-PET and CT read side by side
- Optimized PET/CT protocol

- *Breathing*
- *Contrast agents*
- Summary
- References

Lung cancer is the leading cause of tumor-related deaths [1]. Although rates of bronchial carcinoma–related death in men have decreased on average by 1.8% annually during the past decade, the incidence of lung cancer in women is increasing [1]. Non–small cell lung cancer (NSCLC) accounts for approximately 80% of bronchogenic malignancies. Among the 150 factors that help determine NSCLC prognosis, the tumor stage, as defined by the American Joint Committee on Cancer is considered to be the most important [2,3]. Thus, the choice of therapy options, including surgery, radiation therapy, and chemotherapy—used alone or in combination [4,5]—is based on the tumor stage. Consequently, the accurate determination of tumor size, potential infiltration of adjacent structures, mediastinal lymph node involvement, and the detection of distant metastases are of central importance. Especially the diagnosis of contralateral lymph node metastases and distant metastases is crucial (stage IIIB and stage V) as these exclude a curative therapeutic approach [6].

In general, morphological imaging with CT is the method of choice to define the extent of the primary tumor and to assess the tumor. However, one of the main limitations of CT is that it has a low accuracy when differentiating benign from malignant lymph nodes using a size criterion of 1 cm for mediastinal nodes and 7 mm for hilar nodes [7–9]. The limitations of this size-based node characterization system is well documented: up to 21% of nodes smaller than 10 mm are malignant, whereas 40% of nodes larger than 10 mm are benign [8–11].

In contrast, metabolic imaging using fluorine-18-2-fluoro-2-deoxy-D-glucose (FDG) positron emission tomography (PET) has been shown to be substantially more sensitive and specific in the detection and characterization of metastases to mediastinal lymph nodes (Fig. 1). Several studies compared the accuracy of CT and FDG-PET [6,11–14]: in

a Department of Nuclear Medicine, University of Duisburg, Hufelandstrasse 55 D-45122, Essen, Germany
b Department of Diagnostic and Interventional Radiology, University of Duisburg, Hufelandstrasse 55, D-45122 Essen, Germany
* Corresponding author.
E-mail address: lutz.freudenberg@uni-essen.de (L.S. Freudenberg).

1556-8598/07/$ – see front matter © 2007 Elsevier Inc. All rights reserved.
pet.theclinics.com

doi:10.1016/j.cpet.2006.09.001

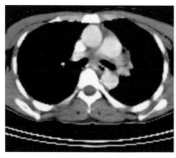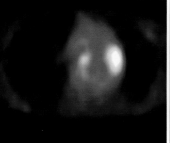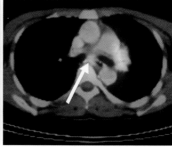

Fig. 1. CT (*left*), FDG-PET (*middle*), and FDG-PET/CT (*right*) of a 49-year-old male with diagnosis of NSCLC before neoadjuvant combined radiotherapy/chemotherapy. CT and FDG-PET clearly visualize a vital hilar metastasis. FDG-PET additionally shows additional tracer-uptake mediastinally. Exact localization is difficult due to little anatomic detail, CT alone is ambiguous. Integrated FDG-PET/CT allows diagnosis of a vital infracarinal metastasis (*arrow*).

a meta-analysis on staging lung cancer with PET and CT, Dwamena and colleagues [11] concluded that FDG-PET was significantly more accurate than CT and reported sensitivity and specificity values of 79% and 91% for PET and 60% and 77% for CT, respectively. Weber and colleagues [6], in a recent meta-analysis according to the Agency for Health Care Policy Research criteria, reported a significantly increased sensitivity and specificity of FDG-PET compared with CT in assessment of mediastinal lymph nodes and distant metastases with a sensitivity of 83% (95% CI: 75%–89%), and 96% (95% CI: 89%–99%), respectively. Based on FDG-PET findings, 18% of the patients received a different therapy compared with CT [6].

On the other hand, limited anatomic information in FDG-PET images frequently renders localization of a lesion and its potential infiltration into adjacent organs difficult [15,16]. Thus, for maximal diagnostic benefit, functional data sets should be read in conjunction with morphologic images. Image fusion and side-by-side image evaluation of morphologic and functional data sets have been proposed [17]. However, differences in patient positioning and motion-induced data misregistration cause image fusion of separately acquired CT and PET image sets to be complex and often unsatisfactory [18,19]. This limitation can be overcome by collecting functional and morphologic data in one examination. The availability of dual-modality PET/CT tomographs provides the technical basis for intrinsically aligned functional and morphologic data sets [19].

The purpose of this article is to summarize the accuracy of dual-modality FDG-PET/CT imaging in staging of NSCLC as compared with FDG-PET alone, and with FDG-PET as well as CT read side by side. Furthermore, an optimized PET/CT protocol for patients who have lung cancer is outlined.

FDG-PET/CT versus FDG-PET

Several studies have reported a higher sensitivity of FDG-PET/CT compared with FDG-PET alone.

For tumor staging, the sole use of conventional FDG-PET is limited based on the limited anatomical data. Thus, tumor size and a potential infiltration may be difficult to assess on PET alone. It has been shown in recent studies that in tumor staging of patients who have lung cancer, analysis of integrated FDG-PET/CT images is superior to that of FDG-PET or CT images alone when assessing the tumor stage [20–23]. The integration of morphologic CT and functional PET data sets particularly enables the most accurate differentiation of viable tumor tissue relative to all adjacent structures (eg, differentiation of tumor from atelectasis, detection of focal chest wall infiltration or mediastinal invasion) (Fig. 2) [20–22,24].

Furthermore, PET/CT resulted in further improvement of N staging compared with PET alone due to the ability to reveal the exact location of metastatic lymph nodes: accurate anatomic correlation is of benefit for exact localization of a solitary

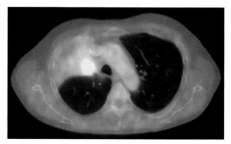

Fig. 2. FDG-PET/CT of a 47-year-old male with diagnosis of NSCLC before first treatment. Integrated FDG-PET/CT enables the most accurate differentiation of viable tumor tissue relative to atelectasis.

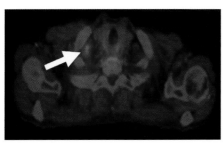

Fig. 3. FDG-PET/CT of a 54-year-old male with NSCLC (pancoast-tumor) showing a supraclavicular lymph node metastasis 0.5 cm in diameter not visible in CT alone and unambiguous in FDG-PET.

lymph node metastasis and thus allows exact classification as N1 or N2 disease, which is difficult but important [25]. Furthermore, FDG-PET/CT is important when identifying supraclavicular N3 disease (Fig. 3) [20,22,23,26]. Results of recent studies with respect to the tumor–node–metastasis (TNM) system are summarized in Table 1. These studies reported significant advantages of FDG-PET/CT compared with FDG-PET alone.

It is generally concluded that dual-modality PET/CT represents the most efficient and accurate approach to NSCLC staging, with a profound effect on therapy and, hence, patient prognosis [20,22,23,26,27]. Antoch and colleagues [26] described that PET/CT findings led to a change in tumor stage in 26% of patients compared with PET data alone, resulting in a change of treatment plans in 15%. Cerfolio and colleagues [20], Lardinois and colleagues [22], and Aquino and colleagues [23] likewise found tumor staging was significantly more accurate with integrated PET-CT than with PET alone, especially for stage I and stage II (see Table 1) [20,22,23,26,27].

In conclusion, dual-modality FDG-PET/CT data enabled more accurate staging of NSCLC than either FDG-PET or CT, reflecting the inherent limitations of these two imaging modalities when used alone. However, as Buell and colleagues [24] argue, the somewhat unrealistic comparisons of FDG-PET alone with integrated FDG-PET/CT must show an advantage for FDG-PET/CT. To allow for a more balanced study design that reflects clinical reality, FDG-PET/CT must be compared with a side-by-side evaluation of conventional FDG-PET and CT scans.

FDG-PET/CT versus FDG-PET and CT read side by side

In general, visual correlation of CT and FDG-PET improves interpretation of both datasets [24,28]. For image coregistration, computer-assisted support appears helpful. However, in clinical practice, routine acceptance of retrospective image fusion may be limited by the complexity of retrospective coregistration algorithms and their limited accuracy for aligning areas of interest in independently acquired scans. Nonlinear registration techniques are required to account for complex patient motion, especially in the thorax and upper abdomen [29].

Several investigators have studied the impact of software image fusion in NSCLC showing significant improvement in staging of fused CT and FDG-PET data compared with FDG-PET alone [21,23,24,30]. However, Vansteenkiste and colleagues [30] reported no significant differences between image fusion of FDG-PET and CT data compared with visual correlation. Halpern and colleagues [21] as well as Buell and colleagues [24]

Table 1: Sensitivity of FDG-PET versus FDG-PET/CT with respect to TNM and overall tumor staging (I–IV) according to American Joint Committee on Cancer

Study	Patients	TNM	FDG-PET	FDG-PET/CT	P value
Cerfolio et al [20]	129	T	38%–70%	50%–100%	.001
		N	60%–80%	77%–92%	.008
		M	81%–82%	90%–92%	NS
		Overall staging	17%–83%	50%–94%	NR
Halpern et al [21]	36	T	67%	97%	<.05
		Overall staging	57%	83%	<.05
Lardinois et al [22]	50	N	49%	93%	.013
		Overall staging	40%	88%	.001
Aquino et al [23]	45	N	59%–76%	71%–76%	.01
		Overall staging	53%–62%	73%–76%	.002
Antoch et al [26]	27	Overall staging	74%	96%	<.05
Shim et al [27]	106	N	–	85%	–
Keidar et al [31]	42	Restaging	96%	96%	NS

Abbreviations: NR, not reported; NS, not significant.

describe advantages of software fusion with regard to the T stage and the N stage when compared with FDG-PET alone.

Lardinois and colleagues [22] reported significant advantages of FDG-PET/CT over FDG-PET and CT read side by side when examining 50 patients who have surgically staged NSCLC. They report a diagnostic accuracy for integrated FDG-PET/CT and visual correlation of FDG-PET and CT of 89% and 77%, respectively. This difference was statistically significant. Furthermore, they found additional information by FDG-PET/CT in 41% of their patients. However, as Buell and colleagues [24] note, this advantage of PET/CT was achieved by evaluating a multitude of different parameters, some of which were only of limited clinical relevance. Keidar and colleagues [31] performed a study addressing the diagnostic value of FDG-PET/CT versus FDG-PET and CT read side by side in suspected lung cancer recurrence showing no differences in sensitivity. Although FDG-PET/CT performed better with respect to specificity and positive predictive values, these results did not reach the level of statistical significance.

Two recent studies evaluated the accuracy of PET/CT and included oncology patients who have different malignancies. Their results are of interest with respect to NSCLC, because patients who have lung cancer represent the largest patient cohort within both patient populations. Antoch and colleagues [32] evaluated FDG-PET/CT for tumor staging in 260 patients who have solid tumors (57 patients who have NSCLC) and conclude that FDG-PET/CT is able to detect significantly more lesions than FDG-PET or CT alone. Based on a change in the TNM stage, they reported a change in patient management in 6% of patients who have FDG-PET/CT compared with FDG-PET and CT evaluated side by side. Buell and colleagues [24] evaluated side-by-side analysis of CT and conventional FDG-PET in 733 patients (174 who have bronchial cancer) with respect to patient groups that may benefit the most from the integrated PET/CT scanners. They showed that side-by-side reading of FDG-PET and CT failed to yield conclusive data with regard to lesion characterization in only 7.4% of patients so FDG-PET/CT might have been helpful in these cases.

Until now, only one study has evaluated the differences of integrated FDG-PET/CT versus software-based image fusion in NSCLC. Halpern and colleagues [21] reported equal results with regard to the T stage and the N stage for image fusion and PET/CT in cases in which software fusion was successful. However, software fusion of separately obtained PET and CT studies was successful in only 68% of the patients and failed in 32%. As stated by the authors, the performance of software fusion can significantly be improved when including transmission PET scans to a success rate from approximately 70% to 95% [33].

Further studies will have to evaluate the impact of integrated FDG-PET/CT versus software fusion keeping in mind that misregistration is not totally avoidable even with a combined PET/CT scanner [34,35]. Finally, the actual impact of more accurate tumor staging—beyond therapeutic decision making—on patient survival will have to be determined in future studies.

Optimized PET/CT protocol

Local misregistration between the CT and the PET in integrated PET/CT and the use of CT contrast media may bias the PET tracer distribution following CT-based attenuation correction [36]. Consequently, protocol requirements for PET/CT with diagnostic CT include alternative contrast application schemes to handle CT contrast agents appropriately. In addition, a special breathing protocol can avoid motion-induced artifacts in the area of the diaphragm. Using an optimized acquisition protocol significantly improves integrated PET/CT imaging and thus can further improve staging of NSCLC.

Breathing

The coregistration accuracy in combined PET/CT imaging is mainly impaired by respiration-induced mismatches between the CT and the PET. These artifacts are particularly severe when standard breath-hold techniques (eg, scanning at maximum inspiration) are transferred directly from clinical CT to combined PET/CT without further adaptation [34]. Goerres and colleagues [37] investigated the misregistration of pulmonary lesions with a combined PET/CT system and detected the mismatch between PET and CT to be most severe if the CT was performed during maximal inspiration of the patient. The registration error was found to be in the range of 5 to 33 mm in this setting [37,38]. Combined PET/CT scans during normal respiration go along with respiration artifacts in the majority of cases as well. To reduce potential misregistration from differences in the breathing pattern between two complementary PET and CT data sets, our protocol uses a limited breath-hold technique: patients are asked to hold their breath in normal expiration only for the time that the CT takes to cover the lower lung and liver, which is typically less than 15 seconds. Instructing the patient before the PET/CT examinations on the breath-hold command is essential in avoiding serious respiration artifacts [39]. When applying the limited breath-hold technique, the frequency of severe artifacts in the area of the diaphragm was reduced by half, and the spatial extent of respiration-induced artifacts can be reduced by at least 40% compared with the acquisition protocols without any breathing instructions [39].

With the introduction of multirow CT technology of up to 64 detector rows into PET/CT designs, the incidence of respiration artifacts in PET/CT examinations can further be reduced. This applies also to patients who are unable to follow any breath-hold instructions. For PET/CT imaging of normally breathing patients, a substantial improvement of image quality can be expected from employing CT technology with six or more detector rows as respiration-induced artifacts are reduced in both magnitude and prominence [38,40]. In conclusion, special breathing protocols are effective and should be used for CT scans as part of combined imaging protocols in dual-modality PET/CT.

Contrast agents

Standard application of intravenous CT contrast agents in combined PET/CT may lead to high-density artifacts on CT and attenuation-corrected PET [35]. To avoid associated diagnostic pitfalls, a special contrast injection protocol is needed. Comparing different protocols, Beyer and colleagues [41] found a reproducible high image quality in the CT image and in the attenuation-corrected PET image without high-density image artifacts when using a dual-phase injection (80 and 60 mL at 3 and 1.5 mL/s, respectively) of contrast agent in the caudocranial direction with a 50-second delay.

Summary

Software coregistration of FDG-PET and CT datasets as well as integrated FDG-PET/CT enable significantly more accurate assessment of NSCLC staging than either modality alone. Integrated FDG-PET/CT has been shown to be more accurate in NSCLC staging than FDG-PET and CT read side by side. However, the benefits of anatometabolic imaging using FDG-PET/CT can only be fully exploited if optimized acquisition protocols are implemented.

References

[1] Jemal A, Thomas A, Murray T, et al. Cancer statistics, 2002. CA Cancer J Clin 2002;52:23–47.

[2] Brundage MD, Davies D, Mackillop WJ. Prognostic factors in non-small cell lung cancer: a decade of progress. Chest 2002;122:1037–57.

[3] Greene FL, Page DL, Fleming ID, et al. AJCC cancer staging manual. 6th edition. New York: Springer; 2002.

[4] Smythe WR. Treatment of stage I and II non-small cell lung cancer. Cancer Control 2001;8: 318–25.

[5] Haura EB. Treatment of advanced nonsmall cell lung cancer: a review of current randomised clinical trials and an examination of emerging therapies. Cancer Control 2001;8: 326–36.

[6] Weber WA, Dietlein M, Hellwig D, et al. PET with (18)F-fluorodeoxyglucose for staging of non-small cell lung cancer. Nuklearmedizin 2003; 42:135–44.

[7] Glazer GM, Gross BH, Quint LE, et al. Normal mediastinal lymph nodes: number and size according to American Thoracic Society mapping. AJR Am J Roentgenol 1985;144:261–5.

[8] Lowe VJ, DeLong DM, Hoffman JM, et al. Optimum scanning protocol for FDGPET evaluation of pulmonary malignancy. J Nucl Med 1995;36: 883–7.

[9] Deslauriers J, Gregoire J. Clinical and surgical staging of non-small cell lung cancer. Chest 2000;117:96S–103S.

[10] Staples CA, Muller NL, Miller RR, et al. Mediastinal nodes in bronchogenic carcinoma: comparison between CT and mediastinoscopy. Radiology 1988;167:367–72.

[11] Dwamena BA, Sonnad SS, Angobaldo JO, et al. Metastases from non-small cell lung cancer: mediastinal staging in the 1990s–meta-analytic comparison of PET and CT. Radiology 1999; 213:530–6.

[12] Adams S, Baum RP, Stuckensen T, et al. Prospective comparison of 18F-FDG PET with conventional imaging modalities (CT, MRI, US) in lymph node staging of head and neck cancer. Eur J Nucl Med 1998;25: 1255–60.

[13] Marom EM, McAdams HP, Erasmus JJ, et al. Staging non-small cell lung cancer with whole-body PET. Radiology 1999;212:803–9.

[14] van Tinteren H, Hoekstra OS, Smit EF, et al. Effectiveness of positron emission tomography in the preoperative assessment of patients with suspected non-small-cell lung cancer: the PLUS multicentre randomised trial. Lancet 2002;359: 1388–93.

[15] Diederichs CG, Staib L, Vogel J, et al. Values and limitations of 18F-fluorodeoxyglucosepositron-emission tomography with preoperative evaluation of patients with pancreatic masses. Pancreas 2000;20:109–16.

[16] Weber WA, Avril N, Schwaiger M. Relevance of positron emission tomography (PET) in oncology. Strahlenther Onkol 1999;175: 356–73.

[17] Wahl RL, Quint LE, Cieslak RD, et al. "Anatometabolic" tumor imaging: fusion of FDG PET with CT or MRI to localize foci of increased activity. J Nucl Med 1993;34:1190–7.

[18] Townsend DW. A combined PET/CT scanner: the choices. J Nucl Med 2001;42:533–4.

[19] Beyer T, Townsend DW, Blodgett TM. Dual-modality PET/CT tomography for clinical oncology. Q J Nucl Med 2002;46:24–34.

[20] Cerfolio RJ, Ojha B, Bryant AS, et al. The accuracy of integrated PET-CT compared with dedicated PET alone for the staging of patients with nonsmall cell lung cancer. Ann Thorac Surg 2004;78:1017–23.

[21] Halpern BS, Schiepers C, Weber WA, et al. Presurgical staging of non-small cell lung cancer: positron emission tomography, integrated positron emission tomography/CT, and software image fusion. Chest 2005;128:2289–97.

[22] Lardinois D, Weder W, Hany TF, et al. Staging of non-small-cell lung cancer with integrated positron-emission tomography and computed tomography. N Engl J Med 2003;19:2500–7.

[23] Aquino SL, Asmuth JC, Alpert NM, et al. Improved radiologic staging of lung cancer with 2-[18F]-fluoro-2-deoxy-D-glucose-positron emission tomography and computed tomography registration. J Comput Assist Tomogr 2003; 27:479–84.

[24] Buell U, Wieres FJ, Schneider W, et al. 18FDG-PET in 733 consecutive patients with or without side-by-side CT evaluation: analysis of 921 lesions. Nuklearmedizin 2004;43:210–6.

[25] Asamura H, Suzuki K, Kondo H, et al. Where is the boundary between N1 and N2 stations in lung cancer? Ann Thorac Surg 2000;70:1839–45.

[26] Antoch G, Stattaus J, Nemat AT, et al. Non-small cell lung cancer: dual-modality PET/CT in preoperative staging. Radiology 2003;229:526–33.

[27] Shim SS, Lee KS, Kim BT, et al. Non-small cell lung cancer: prospective comparison of integrated FDG PET/CT and CT alone for preoperative staging. Radiology 2005;236:1011–9.

[28] Reinartz P, Wieres FJ, Schneider W, et al. Side-by-side reading of PET and CT scans in oncology: which patients might profit from integrated PET/CT? Eur J Nucl Med Mol Imaging 2004;31: 1456–61.

[29] Hutton BF, Braun M. Software for image registration: algorithms, accuracy, efficacy. Sem Nucl Med 2003;33:180–92.

[30] Vansteenkiste JF, Stroobants SG, Dupont PJ, et al. FDG-PET scan in potentially operable non-small cell lung cancer: do anatometabolic PET-CT fusion images improve the localisation of regional lymph node metastases? The Leuven Lung Cancer Group. Eur J Nucl Med 1998;25:1495–501.

[31] Keidar Z, Haim N, Guralnik L, et al. PET/CT using 18F-FDG in suspected lung cancer recurrence: diagnostic value and impact on patient management. J Nucl Med 2004;45:1640–6.

[32] Antoch G, Saoudi N, Kuehl H, et al. Accuracy of whole-body dual-modality fluorine-18-2-fluoro-2-deoxy-D-glucose positron emission tomography and computed tomography (FDG-PET/CT) for tumor staging in solid tumors: comparison with CT and PET. J Clin Oncol 2004;22:4357–68.

[33] Slomka PJ, Dey D, Przetak C, et al. Automated 3-dimensional registration of stand-alone (18)F-FDG whole-body PET with CT. J Nucl Med 2003; 44:1156–67.

[34] Beyer T, Antoch G, Muller S, et al. Acquisition protocol considerations for combined PET/CT imaging. J Nucl Med 2004;45(Suppl 1):25S–35S.

[35] Cohade C, Osman M, Marshall LN, et al. PET-CT: accuracy of PET and CT spatial registration of lung lesions. Eur J Nucl Med Mol Imaging 2003;30:721–6.

[36] Antoch G, Freudenberg LS, Egelhof T, et al. Focal tracer uptake: a potential artifact in contrast-enhanced dual-modality PET/CT scans. J Nucl Med 2002;43:1339–42.

[37] Goerres GW, Burger C, Schwitter MR, et al. PET/CT of the abdomen: optimizing the patient breathing pattern. Eur Radiol 2003;13:734–9.

[38] Goerres GW, Kamel E, Heidelberg TN, et al. PET/CT image co-registration in the thorax: influence of respiration. Eur J Nucl Med Mol Imaging 2002;29:351–60.

[39] Beyer T, Antoch G, Blodgett T, et al. Dual-modality PET/CT imaging: the effect of respiratory motion on combined image quality in clinical oncology. Eur J Nucl Med Mol Imaging 2003;30:588–96.

[40] Beyer T, Rosenbaum S, Veit P, et al. Respiration artifacts in whole-body (18)F-FDG PET/CT studies with combined PET/CT tomographs employing spiral CT technology with 1 to 16 detector rows. Eur J Nucl Med Mol Imaging 2005;32:1429–39.

[41] Beyer T, Antoch G, Bockisch A, et al. Optimized intravenous contrast administration for diagnostic whole-body 18F-FDG PET/CT. J Nucl Med 2005;46:429–35.

POSITRON
EMISSION
TOMOGRAPHY

PET Clin 1 (2007) 353–355

Index

Note: Page numbers of article titles are in **boldface** type.

A

Adenocarcinoma, spiculation of, 295
Air bronchography, 295
Arteriovenous fistulas, 294
Aspergilloma, 294
Atelectasis, 294
Attenuation, 293

B

Bayesian analysis, of pulmonary nodules, 297
Biopsy, of lung nodule, 298, 308
Breathing, in PET
    for radiation therapy planning, 322
    versus PET/CT, 350–351
Bronchography, air, 295
Brown fat, FDG uptake in, 311

C

Calcification, 291–292
Cancer, lung. *See* Lung cancer.
Cavitation, 295–296
Central calcification pattern, 291
CHART (continuous hyperfractionated accelerated
    radiotherapy), 324–325
Chest radiography, 290
Computed tomography, in lung cancer, **289–300**.
    See also PET/CT, in lung cancer.
    attenuation in, 293
    Bayesian analysis of, 297
    calcification in, 291–292
    cavitation in, 295–296
    clinical history and, 289–290
    dynamic enhancement in, 292
    follow-up evaluation in, 297–298
    for needle biopsy, 298
    for radiation therapy planning, 318–322
    for staging, 303–308

    growth rate of, 296
    margins in, 294–295
    morphology of, 293–294
    nodule location and, 291
    number of nodules in, 291
    size of lesions in, 291
Continuous hyperfractionated accelerated
    radiotherapy (CHART), 324–325
Contrast agents
    for CT, 292
    for PET/CT, 351
    for radiation therapy planning, 324–325
    for staging, 301
Cost analysis, definition of, 340
Cost-benefit analysis, definition of, 340
Cost-effectiveness, of PET
    in non–small cell lung cancer, **329–337**
    in pulmonary nodule characterization, **339–346**
    methods of, 340–342
    overview of, 339–340
Cost-minimization study, definition of, 340
Cost-utility analysis, definition of, 340

D

Decision-modeling, for PET cost-effectiveness,
    331–332
Diffuse calcification pattern, 291

E

Eccentric calcification, 291
Embolism, pulmonary, 294

F

Fine needle biopsy, of lung nodule, 298, 308
Fistulas, arteriovenous, 294
^{18}F-Fluoro-azomycin arabinoside, as lung cancer
    tracer, 325

doi:10.1016/S1556-8598(07)00013-2

Moving?

Make sure your subscription moves with you!

To notify us of your new address, find your **Clinics Account Number** (located on your mailing label above your name), and contact customer service at:

E-mail: elspcs@elsevier.com

800-654-2452 (subscribers in the U.S. & Canada)
407-345-4000 (subscribers outside of the U.S. & Canada)

Fax number: 407-363-9661

Elsevier Periodicals Customer Service
6277 Sea Harbor Drive
Orlando, FL 32887-4800

*To ensure uninterrupted delivery of your subscription, please notify us at least 4 weeks in advance of move.

ELSEVIER